Restful Insights to Achieving Deeper Sleep with One Powerful Guided Meditation to Fall Asleep

MINDFUL SLUMBER

A Simple Guide to Better Sleep Through Guided Meditation

ZACH STEIN

Publisher: Seaglow Publishing

Audio version features: A Tranquil Lullaby on Acoustic Guitar with 528 Hz Binaural Beats

Note: This is meant to be a companion to the audio book.

Dedication

The meditations provided in this book are intended for relaxation and sleep enhancement purposes only. They are not a substitute for professional medical advice, diagnosis, or treatment. The author of this book is not a licensed physician or healthcare professional.

If you are experiencing chronic insomnia, depression, or any other medical condition, or if you have feelings of suicide, it is important to seek help from a qualified physician or healthcare provider. Do not disregard professional medical advice or delay seeking it because of anything you have read in this book.

The home remedies and techniques mentioned in this book are provided for informational purposes only, and their effectiveness may vary from person to person. Individual results cannot be guaranteed. Always consult with a healthcare professional before starting any new treatment or making changes to your health care routine.

By using this book, you acknowledge and agree that you are doing so at your own risk and that the author and publisher are not liable for any direct, indirect, incidental, consequential, or punitive damages arising from your use of the information contained herein.

The meditations in this book are designed to be relaxing and calming, providing a peaceful escape from the stresses of daily life. If you are listening to the audio version of this book, please ensure your safety by not listening while driving or operating heavy machinery.

All publications and brands mentioned within this book are the property of their respective owners. All rights, copyrights, and trademarks belong to their respective holders. The mention of any

Contents

1

Preface

Are sleepless nights tormenting your life, leaving you exhausted and drained? Do you lie awake, tossing and turning, as anxiety and frustration envelop you in the darkness? Insomnia can be relentless, affecting your mood, energy, and overall well-being.

There was a time when I couldn't even imagine falling asleep peacefully. It was a never-ending battle every night. I'd lay in bed, staring at the ceiling for hours on end. My mind raced with worries and anxieties. It was like my brain had a mind of its own, and it chose the worst possible time to go into overdrive.

Sound frustrating? It was beyond frustrating. It was like a cycle of misery. The more I tried to sleep, the harder it became. I felt exhausted all the time, but sleep just eluded me.

For me it wasn't just the exhaustion that struck me, but it was also the sheer helplessness of it all. As I'd lie there, eyes heavy with fatigue, the prospect of sleep would seem miles away. Minutes would feel like hours, and the night would stretch on seemingly with no end. Each tick of the clock was a cruel reminder of how elusive rest had become.

But the toll of insomnia went beyond just those sleepless nights. It crept into every aspect of my life, affecting my family and work in ways I couldn't have imagined. At home, I'd be irritable and short-tempered, unable to muster the energy to engage with loved ones or enjoy quality time together. The frustration from sleepless nights would spill over into my interactions, leaving me feeling disconnected and distant from the people I cared about most.

And at work, it was like a silent saboteur. The lack of sleep would sap my focus and concentration, making even the simplest tasks feel like insurmountable obstacles. My productivity plummeted, and I'd find myself struggling to meet deadlines and perform at my best. It was a vicious cycle—lack of sleep leading to decreased performance, which in turn fueled my anxiety about work, further exacerbating my insomnia.

I'd often find myself in a constant state of fatigue, trying to hide the dark circles under my eyes and the mental fog that clouded my thoughts during meetings and projects. The fear of making mistakes haunted me, and it became a self-fulfilling prophecy as my sleep deprivation continued to take its toll.

The impact on my family and work life was undeniable, and it was heart-wrenching to witness. I'd see the concern in the eyes of my loved ones and the frustration of my colleagues, who couldn't fully understand what I was going through. It felt like I was letting everyone down, including myself.

And I tried everything—every trick, remedy, and old wives' tale that promised a shred of hope. Warm milk before bed? Check. Lavender-scented pillows? Of course. Counting sheep until I lost count? Absolutely. But the cruel irony was that these supposed solutions only seemed to mock me further.

Desperation led me down some strange paths too. I remember that one infamous night when I convinced myself that wearing a pair of warm socks filled with mustard powder would be the key to unlocking sleep's embrace. Yes, you heard that right, mustard socks. It was a bizarre concoction I'd read about on a forum. Needless to say, I woke up with mustard-stained sheets and the same exhaustion that had become my constant companion.

I'd also tried some well-known false remedies that promised instant relief. The so-called "miracle" sleep pills, advertised on late-night TV infomercials, made grandiose claims but left me feeling groggy and disoriented, with no real improvement in my sleep quality. And don't get me started on the infamous "cabbage pillow" trend that briefly swept through social media. I spent a night with a cabbage tucked under my pillow, and all I got was a peculiar odor and an even greater sense of disillusionment.

Each failed attempt was a reminder of the relentless grip insomnia had on me. It was as if the more I sought a solution, the more elusive sleep became. It was a maddening cycle of trial and error that left me feeling defeated and, at times, utterly ridiculous.

But I suppose that's the nature of insomnia—it makes you willing to try anything, no matter how outlandish, just for the chance of a few moments of rest. It's a testament to the lengths we'll go to escape the torment of sleeplessness, even if it means donning mustard socks or sharing our bed with a head of cabbage.

Does this feel familiar to you? The tossing, the turning, the itchy dry red eyes? It's a tormenting dance that so many of us suffering from insomnia know all too well.

But then, one day, my life took an unexpected turn. I met someone who had been through the same sleepless nights and relentless battles with insomnia. They showed me the power of meditation in a way I had never experienced before, a step by step method that held the promise of actual relief.

With this methodology, I found something I had longed for—a path to tranquility. The power of meditation wasn't just in its promise; it was in its practice. Night after night, I followed this routine, and slowly but surely, the dance of sleeplessness began to change its rhythm.

My restless mind, which had once been my greatest adversary, started to cooperate. The hours of endless tossing and turning began to dwindle. Instead of counting the minutes, I counted the moments of serenity that meditation brought me.

Of course, it wasn't a magical cure, but a piece to the puzzle. Insomnia still visited from time to time, but it no longer held me captive. Meditation became my ally, my refuge in the darkness of sleepless nights. It gave me the power to reclaim my nights and find solace in the embrace of slumber.

So, if you're out there, battling insomnia's relentless grip, know that there is a way—a path to peaceful sleep that doesn't involve mustard socks or cabbage pillows. It starts with setting the stage, breathing mindfully, scanning your body, and immersing yourself in a tranquil world of your own creation. It's a journey worth taking, one breath at a time.

2

Introduction

Congratulations on taking this crucial step towards prioritizing yourself! In the relentless hustle of life, carving out these sacred moments of 'me-time' is a testament to your commitment to self-care. By embarking on this journey, you're not only saying 'yes' to relaxation but also to a deeper understanding of your own needs and desires.

When insomnia takes hold, the persistent feeling of fatigue becomes a constant shadow, with sluggishness lingering through each hour of the day. Concentration falters, tasks that require focus become herculean, and irritability creeps into interactions, making small frustrations feel insurmountable. Sleep deprivation may lead to mood swings with peaks of okayness that plummet into valleys of overwhelm without warning. Productivity often wanes as memory plays tricks, hiding away important details and tasks.

Without sleep the body breaks down, and may signal distress with headaches or an uneasy stomach, while a once robust defense against colds and infections weakens. As night falls, the irony of insomnia strikes; the deep tiredness doesn't translate to sleep. Instead, there's the lying awake, eyes wide in the dark, or the frequent interruptions of rest that no amount of tossing and turning can mend, only to be followed by the frustration of waking, with the night's rest feeling incomplete.

If you find yourself wrestling with the relentless restlessness of insomnia, know that you're not alone, nor is it a reflection of any failing on your part. It's not your fault. Many people will encounter bouts of sleeplessness at some stage in their lives, a common thread in the human existence is that sleep depravation is often tied to factors beyond your control.

Insomnia can be the body's alarm bell, signaling anything from transient stress to underlying health issues that may require attention. It's a condition that does not discriminate, touching the lives of countless individuals across the spectrum of age and circumstance. So, when the silence of the night is broken by the ticking of the clock, or a dripping faucet, remember that this is a shared experience, one that speaks not of personal fault but rather the intricate and sometimes challenging nature of our biological rhythms and health.

Think of this guided meditation for better sleep as your personal vacation, a retreat from the cacophony of daily commitments, where the sole agenda is your well-being. Remember, by investing time in yourself, you're not only fostering personal growth but also rejuvenating your health, spirit, and energy. Here's to you and this wonderful act of self-love!

Hello and welcome to this special self-care session of guided meditation designed specifically to lead you into a profound and restorative night of sleep. Relax and let's begin this guided meditation and tranquil journey to better sleep.

3

About This Meditation

We spend approximately a third of our lives sleeping, yet so many of us struggle to truly achieve that rejuvenating rest we so deeply crave. Sleep is essential for our wellbeing—it recharges our mind, repairs our body, and revitalizes our spirit.

If you find yourself listening to this, I want you to know that it's perfectly okay to seek assistance in achieving deeper sleep. Whether you're here for yourself, or perhaps thinking about the wellbeing of a family member, or even your newborn, know that sleep challenges are shared by many.

Stress and anxiety, the burdens of our daily life, can often be core culprits behind our sleep disturbances. It isn't your fault. These feelings are natural and are experienced by countless individuals across the globe.

But for this moment, I invite you to release the weight of the day, to let go of the mental and emotional baggage, and to sink into a peaceful slumber.

In the background, you can hear the gentle strumming of a guitar, playing a soft lullaby designed to soothe your soul and lull you into sleep. Allow the music to envelop you, creating a cocoon of tranquility around you.

As we embark on this guided journey together, keep in mind that your only responsibility in this moment is to relax and allow yourself to be guided. There is no right or wrong way to meditate; it's all about finding what feels right for you.

Though before we dive deeper, take a moment to get comfortable in your chosen space. Ensure you're in a position where you can truly relax, whether that's lying down or sitting up with support. Allow the soft lullaby to wash over you, signaling to your body and mind that it's time to unwind.

Sleep is a foundational pillar of our wellbeing—it recharges our mind, mends our body, and revitalizes our spirit. Yet, many of us, for various reasons, find that deep, rejuvenating sleep elusive.

If you're here, know that sleep challenges are a shared experience. Whether it's for you, a family member, or even your newborn, you're not alone in this. Our modern world with its myriad stresses and anxieties often stands in the way of a peaceful slumber. But remember, it's not your fault.

528 Hz Binaural Beats

If you're listening to the audio version of this meditation, in the music of this meditation are interwoven binaural beats—a scientifically backed audio tool that has profound effects on our brain and relaxation states. Binaural beats work by playing slightly different frequencies in each ear. The brain perceives a third tone that is the mathematical difference between the two. It's this third tone that has been shown to have therapeutic qualities.

We've carefully chosen the 528 Hz frequency, a special tone within the Solfeggio frequencies. This frequency, often termed as the 'Love Frequency,' resonates deeply with the heart chakra, ushering in feelings of harmony, love, and compassion. It is known for its profound healing attributes, associated with DNA regeneration and its unique connection to nature.

The ancient solfeggio frequency of 528Hz, the 'Love Frequency,' has been revered for ages for its powerful positive healing qualities. And today, we merge it with Delta Waves, the brainwave state associated with the deepest levels of relaxation and sleep.

Let this combination be your remedy for insomnia. Allow these tones to guide your mind into a realm of deep sleep and rejuvenation. As we embark on this audio journey, feel yourself enveloped in the healing embrace of the 528 Hz frequency, and let it pave the way for a night of transformative sleep.

Mindfulness

This is designed to be a mindfulness meditation because mindful meditations have an intrinsic emphasis on the present moment. Mindfulness, at its core, is the practice of anchoring oneself to the here and now, allowing the individual to become an observer of their thoughts, emotions, and sensations without judgment. This approach can be particularly beneficial for sleep for several reasons.

First, one of the common reasons people find it challenging to fall asleep is because of the ceaseless barrage of thoughts, often revolving around past regrets or anxieties about the future.

Mindfulness addresses this directly by teaching the practitioner to gently acknowledge these thoughts without getting entangled in them. Over time, this practice can reduce the mental noise that often keeps us awake.

Moreover, the relaxation response triggered by mindfulness meditation can counteract the stress response in the body. Chronic stress, characterized by elevated levels of cortisol, can wreak havoc on sleep patterns. Mindfulness helps in reducing this stress response, paving the way for a state of relaxation conducive to deep sleep.

Another advantage of mindfulness for sleep is its emphasis on body awareness. Through mindfulness, individuals can recognize and release areas of physical tension. As the body relaxes, the mind often follows, which can be especially helpful for those who have difficulty disconnecting from the stresses of the day.

Lastly, regular mindfulness practice can improve emotional regulation, reducing instances of mood disorders such as anxiety and depression, both of which can interfere with sleep. By cultivating a non-reactive awareness of one's emotions, it becomes easier to navigate the ebbs and flows of emotional life, which can lead to more consistent, restful nights.

In summary, the decision to use mindfulness guided meditation for better, deeper sleep is anchored in its ability to calm the mind, regulate emotions, and relax the body. Its unique emphasis on present-moment awareness offers a pathway to restful sleep that is both natural and effective.

Mindfulness is a practice of being fully present, of deeply and actively engaging with the now. Mindfulness meditation, distinct from other meditation forms, centers on a keen awareness of what you're sensing and feeling in the present moment. It's not about silencing the mind, but rather observing its nuances without judgment.

Unlike regular meditation, which often involves passive relaxation and perhaps a mantra to guide the mind beyond its chatter, mindfulness meditation invites you to become an active observer. It requires mental discipline, wakefulness, and intention. Both forms, however, share core tenets: the cultivation of kindness, compassion, and being present.

Practicing a mediation style that is mindful may tend to calm the mind, regulate emotions, and relax the body. Its unique emphasis on present-moment awareness offers a pathway to restful sleep that is both natural and effective.

Lullaby

If you're listening to the audio version of this guided meditation, the soft melodies in the background played on acoustic guitars make up a gentle, moving lullaby to lull you into a deep and peaceful sleep.

Lullabies, with their enchanting melodies and tender cadences, have cradled humanity into the realm of sleep for generations. Their ethereal nature has often been described as a bridge between wakefulness and dream, a gentle nudge toward the mysterious abyss of slumber. But what is it about these age-old songs that seem to possess an almost magical ability to coax both the young and old into restful repose?

At the heart of a lullaby lies its simplicity. The melodies are often repetitive, with a rhythm that echoes the comforting beat of a heart. This repetition, akin to a soft, rhythmic rocking, can induce a meditative state, luring the listener deeper into relaxation. The tempo is usually slow, mimicking the pace of breathing when one is at rest, further aligning the body and mind with a state of calm.

Lyrically, lullabies often touch on themes of protection, love, and comfort. Even if the words themselves are not always understood—especially by infants—the soothing tone in which they are sung communicates safety and warmth. The gentle and sometimes familiar melodies can be the most comforting sound, reinforcing a sense of security essential for deep sleep.

Beyond the lyrics and melody, the very structure of lullabies often incorporates descending musical patterns. These patterns can psychologically signal a "letting go" or "winding down," mirroring the descent into sleep. The softness of the notes, the gentle transitions, and the occasional use of white noise-like sounds, such as soft humming or shushing, all contribute to creating an auditory environment that promotes rest.

The true mystery of a lullaby, however, might be in its universality. Across cultures and continents, generations have crafted their own lullabies, each unique but all sharing the same purpose: to beckon the listener into the world of dreams. This universal application speaks to something primal, suggesting that these melodies touch a fundamental part of our human psyche, reminding us of the comforting embrace of a caregiver, the gentle rock of a cradle, and the tranquil world that exists just on the cusp of consciousness.

Meditation

Meditation, with its roots stretching deep into ancient cultures, has been heralded for its manifold benefits in promoting well-being, and among these is its remarkable capacity to enhance deep sleep and fortify self-care. Here's a deeper exploration of how meditation serves these purposes:

A primary reason for sleep disturbances is an overactive mind. Meditation, especially mindfulness-based practices, encourages one to disengage from the continuous stream of thoughts, facilitating a state of calm. Over time, this helps in developing a peaceful mental space conducive to deep sleep.

Progressive relaxation, a feature in many meditation practices, involves focusing on different parts of the body and consciously relaxing them. This not only releases physical tension but also primes the body for restorative sleep.

Chronic stress is known to disrupt sleep patterns and degrade sleep quality. Meditation activates the body's relaxation response, countering the stress response. This balance helps in lowering cortisol levels, making it easier to enter deep sleep phases.

Emotional upheavals can be a barrier to restful sleep. Meditation fosters emotional resilience, equipping individuals to handle their emotions with more grace. As one's emotional landscape becomes steadier, it invariably results in better sleep.

Some studies suggest that regular meditation can boost the production of melatonin, a hormone crucial for regulating sleep-wake cycles.

Meditation nurtures a heightened awareness of one's physical and mental states. This fine-tuned awareness can help individuals recognize patterns or habits that may be detrimental to their sleep, thus allowing for timely intervention.

Breathing practices, often integral to meditation, can help lower heart rate and blood pressure. This physiological shift can aid in preparing the body for deep sleep.

Meditation, by its very nature, is an act of self-care. Setting aside time for introspection and relaxation underscores the importance of looking after oneself. This emphasis on self-care can ripple out, encouraging healthier habits, routines, and attitudes that prioritize one's well-being.

These are the steps we'll follow in today's meditation in a calculated methodology providing a framework to help you have longer, more restful improve sleep.

1. Make a Commitment: Set aside responsibilities and dedicate this time solely for your well-being.
2. Find a Quiet Place: Ensure your surroundings are conducive to relaxation.
3. Get in Position: Sit or lie down comfortably, with your spine aligned.
4. Get Relaxed: Loosen any tight clothing, and let go of physical tension.
5. Focus on Your Breaths: Feel the air entering and leaving your nostrils or mouth. Grounding ourselves with the rhythm of our breath.

6. Guided Imagery: Painting mental pictures to transport you to serene vistas with light breezes, gently swaying trees. Visualizations of a restful sleep..

7. Scan Your Body: Notice any sensations, perhaps tingling or warmth.

8. Awareness of Thoughts: Recognize any thoughts as they arise, without following them. This is sometimes called "Objective Observation" or viewing our thoughts and emotions without judgment, observing the mind as it wanders, without getting caught in its tales. It's a type of "Passive Noticing," embracing the moment without any need to alter it.

9. When the Mind Wanders: Gently bring your attention back to your breath. Continually drawing our attention back to the present.

10. Centering Thoughts: If you get lost, simply return to the here and now.

11. Conclude Gracefully: Give thanks and when you feel ready, gently open your eyes, bringing this heightened awareness into your waking life.

4

Preparation

Before we get started, let's take a few steps to prepare. We'll start by making a commitment, finding a quiet place, and getting into position.

Preparation lays the groundwork for a fruitful meditative experience, much like tilling the soil readies it for sowing seeds. By choosing an appropriate environment, minimizing potential distractions, and adopting a comfortable posture, one establishes a serene external setting. Internally, the value of mindset cannot be overstated.

Approaching meditation with intention, openness, and a non-judgmental attitude creates a receptive mental space, facilitating deeper introspection and connection. This readiness, both external and internal, acts as a beacon, guiding the mind away from the tumult of everyday life and towards the tranquil sanctuaries of inner reflection. It underscores the principle that the quality of one's meditation is often a reflection of the attention given to its antecedent stages.

Commitment

As we continue on this journey towards deep, restorative sleep, I invite you to make a gentle commitment to yourself.

Commitment helps in setting a clear intention. When you make a conscious commitment to meditation, you are signaling to your mind that this is a valuable and important activity. This intentionality can increase the efficacy of the meditation, as it establishes a focused purpose, guiding the mind towards relaxation and deep sleep.

To truly reap the benefits of any meditation practice, creating consistency is key. By committing, you increase the likelihood of practicing regularly, thereby cultivating a routine that allows the body and mind to anticipate and more readily enter a state of relaxation and sleep.

The act of commitment instills discipline. Meditation, especially for beginners, can sometimes be challenging as the mind may wander or resist stillness. A solid commitment provides the necessary discipline to stay the course, even when it feels challenging, ensuring that the practice deepens over time.

Committing to the practice helps to build trust in the process and in oneself. Trusting that mindful meditation will guide you towards better sleep is fundamental for the mind to let go of its guard, allowing the soothing aspects of the meditation to work effectively.

When you commit, you're more likely to prepare adequately by minimizing potential distractions, ensuring a conducive environment for meditation. This might involve turning off electronics, informing family members not to disturb, or choosing a quiet space. Such preparations can significantly enhance the quality of the meditation.

A strong commitment can deepen the experience, leading to more profound immersion in the meditation process. When you fully commit, you allow yourself to be more present, more attuned, and more receptive to the experience, leading to more profound relaxation and a higher likelihood of achieving deep sleep.

In essence, making a commitment serves as the foundational step in a deep sleep mindful meditation, anchoring the practice and paving the way for a transformative experience. Without commitment, the practice may lack depth, consistency, and effectiveness.

Breathe in deeply, filling your lungs with fresh, invigorating air. As you exhale, let go of the day's worries, the to-do lists, and the myriad of thoughts that might be vying for your attention.

Now, in this quiet space, commit to dedicating this time solely for your well-being. Your body, your mind, and your soul deserve this moment of peace, this respite from the hustle and bustle of life. In a world that constantly demands your attention, it's essential to carve out moments like these, where you prioritize yourself.

Imagine wrapping this commitment around you like a soft, warm blanket, providing comfort and assurance. This dedication is a gift you're giving yourself – the gift of tranquility, of serenity, and of deep sleep.

Every breath you take is a reaffirmation of this commitment. Each inhale brings clarity and purpose, and every exhale releases doubts or distractions. By being here, in this moment, you are making a promise to honor, cherish, and care for your well-being.

Let this commitment settle within you, anchoring your intentions and guiding you closer to the peaceful slumber you seek. Remember, by dedicating this time to yourself, you're not only nurturing your body and mind but also ensuring that you wake up refreshed, rejuvenated, and ready to embrace a new day with vitality.

Set Aside Responsibilities

This is a time of self-care. Set aside this time just for you. As a precursor to a successful meditation it is helpful to set our responsibilities and obligations aside for this time. Maybe your parent, caregiver, or have a demanding job. It may feel selfish, but a healthier, refreshed you is a better parent and caregiver to your loved ones, and even a better, more productive provider.

In the tapestry of family life, each thread – every joyous burst of laughter from our children, every soft whisper of a bedtime story – contributes to the richness of our daily existence. Yet, amid the endless dance of parental responsibilities, it's essential to weave in strands of solitude, moments reserved for personal rejuvenation and reflection. This is where meditation, an ancient art of inner harmony, becomes your sanctuary.

As a parent, the concept of uninterrupted serenity might seem as distant as the quiet of dawn in a bustling metropolis. But just as a city sleeps in the wee hours, so too can you find pockets of peace in the dynamic rhythm of family life. To embark on a meditation journey, one must first lay the groundwork for a tranquil mind, and this begins with ensuring that your children are well taken care of in your moments of solitude.

Take time to plan ahead. Like setting stones across a babbling brook to cross with dry feet, arranging care for your children allows you to step into your meditation space with ease. Whether it's coordinating with a partner, scheduling a playdate, or entrusting a grandparent with an hour of storytelling, ensure that your little ones are immersed in an activity that brings them joy and contentment.

Communicate with your family about the significance of this time. Children, even at a tender age, can grasp the concept of 'quiet time'. Share with them that just as they have times for play, learning, and rest, so too do you have a special time to sit quietly and breathe. Let your loved ones know that although you'll be there later, for now this is alone time just for you. In doing so, you're not only setting boundaries, but also teaching them the value of self-care through your example.

The circle of care within our lives often extends beyond the immediate laughter of our children. It may include the comforting embrace of a partner in need of support, the silent strength of aging parents who once cradled us, or even the loyal companionship of pets whose needs speak through actions rather than words. Each of these bonds carries its own set of responsibilities that intertwine deeply with the fabric of our daily lives.

With your spouse, open communication becomes the thread that can weave the tapestry of mutual understanding and support. Share with your partner the importance of your meditation practice, and explore ways you can mutually support each other's pursuit of personal quietude and self-care. It can become a shared journey, a simultaneous solitary retreat, or simply an agreement to hold space for each other's self-care practices.

For aging parents who once acted as our pillars and now lean gently upon us, scheduling becomes an act of love and respect. Consider the rhythms of their day, their medical appointments, their moments of energy, and their stretches of rest. Align your meditation practice with their quietest hours, perhaps during their afternoon nap or while they engage in a hobby they love. Sometimes, the peace needed for your own mindfulness can be found in the calm of their routine.

And let's not forget the pitter-patter of paws, the silent companions who ask for little but give so much. Our pets, sensitive to our emotions and routines, can often sense and respect our need for stillness if we introduce it to them gently. A well-timed walk, a quiet toy, or a cozy nap spot can afford them contentment that aligns with your moments of introspection. Investing in a dog walker for this special time that's just for you may also be an option to consider.

In a world where our work often chases us beyond the confines of office walls, where emails flood in like a relentless tide and the ring of an on-call phone pierces the quiet of the night, the separation between 'work' and 'life' can seem like a blurred line on a worn map. And if you are striving to be the provider, the pressure to sustain and nurture your family can weigh heavily, like an anchor constantly pulling you back to the depths of occupational seas.

In the midst of this, setting boundaries is not just a practice—it's a lifeline. It is about asserting the value of your time and the importance of your mental and emotional space. It's about honoring not just your role as a worker or a provider, but also your inherent worth as an individual. It's about recognizing that to give your best—in every facet of your life—you must also invest in moments of recovery and reflection.

Start by evaluating your work patterns. Identify the true emergencies—the non-negotiables that require your immediate attention—and distinguish them from the perceived urgencies that can, in fact, wait. Convey these boundaries to your boss, with the assurance that clear lines enable you to perform more efficiently when you are on the clock. Honest conversations about workload and expectations can often lead to more sustainable work practices.

Furthermore, embrace the power of 'unplugging'. Carve out deliberate blocks of time where you are unreachable, except for absolute emergencies. Use this time not for idleness, but for activities that replenish your energy, such as meditation. Meditation, in this case, is not an escape from work; it is a strategic retreat—a way to sharpen your mind, to foster resilience, and to emerge more focused and clear-headed.

It's also crucial to create a sanctuary, both physically and mentally. Define a space in your home where work does not intrude, and let this be your meditation haven. Cultivate a mental compartment that is shielded from the tendrils of job-related stress, a psychological 'no-fly zone' from work worries. Within these boundaries, your meditation can flourish, becoming a bulwark against the encroachment of professional demands.

Lastly, embrace the imperfections. There may be days when the arrangements might not go as planned, when the quietude is pierced by a sudden outcry or a pressing need. Approach these moments with grace and understand that meditation is not solely about the absence of noise, but also about the presence of inner calm amidst the chaos. Each day is a fresh opportunity to try again, to negotiate the balance between the roles of caregiver and provider with the role of an individual seeking peace.

In the chapters to follow, we will explore techniques to bring this practice to fruition, even in the liveliest of households. For now, take solace in knowing that with each session of meditation, you're not only nurturing your well-being, but also cultivating a household that values stillness and self-care.

A Quiet Place

Before we dive deeper, take a moment to get comfortable in your chosen space. Ensure you're in a position where you can truly relax, whether that's lying down or sitting up with support. Allow the soft lullaby to wash over you, signaling to your body and mind that it's time to unwind.

Since this is a sleep meditation, your own bed may be the ideal quiet place. But your quiet place also could be any other place you feel safe and comfortable and can be for a while without being disturbed.

Every home, regardless of its size or design, holds unexpected sanctuaries of peace. These nooks, often overlooked in our daily routines, can become ideal spots for sleep meditation or a refreshing nap. For instance, many have found solace in the soft glow of a window sill, especially one that overlooks a garden or a serene landscape. With the gentle hum of nature in the background, a window sill padded with cushions can transform into a meditation retreat or a perfect napping alcove.

Walk-in closets, when decluttered and dimly lit, can also offer an unexpected haven. The insulation provided by clothes makes these spaces unusually quiet, cocooning you in a world detached from the hustle and bustle of the household. Add some soft bedding or a comfortable chair, and you've got a perfect, secluded spot for meditation or rest.

For those with a staircase, the space beneath it often becomes either a storage area or remains unused. However, with a touch of creativity, this area can metamorphose into a cozy hideaway. Some individuals have ingeniously transformed this space, using soft lights, curtains, and plush mats, into their personal relaxation chamber.

Many have rediscovered the nostalgic comfort of building indoor tents or forts using blankets and furniture. This childhood delight, when revisited as an adult, can create a whimsical yet calming space. Draping soft fabrics over chairs or couches, paired with fluffy pillows and fairy lights, can set the scene for a meditative escape or a peaceful nap.

Ultimately, the beauty of finding these unique spots within our homes lies in the joy of rediscovery. It's a testament to the fact that with a bit of imagination, tranquility can be found right where we are.

Another way to go is crafting your own meditation oasis. Creating a personal meditation space is a profound way to honor your commitment to inner peace and personal growth. With a touch of creativity and a few Do It Yourself (DIY) projects, you can design an oasis that resonates with your energy and aesthetic preferences. Here are some DIY ideas to help you craft that perfect space:

1. DIY Water Fountain:

A gentle, trickling water fountain can introduce the calming sound of nature to your meditation space.

- Materials: A small water pump, a basin or bowl, decorative stones, and a waterproof tray or plate.

- Instructions: Place the water pump at the bottom of your basin. Cover it with decorative stones, ensuring the pump's top remains exposed. Fill the basin with water so that it covers the stones but doesn't submerge the pump's top. Once the pump is switched on, water will circulate, creating a soothing water feature.

2. Healing Crystal Garden:

Healing crystals can amplify the energy of your meditation space.

- Materials: A selection of healing crystals (such as amethyst for peace, rose quartz for love, and clear quartz for clarity), a decorative tray or plate, and some sand.
- Instructions: Fill the tray with sand and thoughtfully place your crystals on it. The sand allows you to rearrange your crystals as your energy or intentions change, creating a dynamic, ever-evolving energy landscape.

3. Aromatherapy Diffuser:

Harness the power of essential oils to set the mood for your meditation.

- Materials: A small jar, bamboo skewers or reed sticks, a carrier oil (like almond or safflower), and your choice of essential oil(s).
- Instructions: Fill the jar halfway with the carrier oil, and then add about 20-30 drops of essential oil. Mix well. Place the bamboo skewers or reed sticks into the jar. Over time, the oil will travel up the sticks, diffusing the aroma into your space. You can replenish the mixture as needed.

4. Meditation Cushion:

Create a comfortable seat for your meditation sessions.

- Materials: Fabric of your choice, sewing kit, and stuffing (like cotton batting or buckwheat hulls).
- Instructions: Cut two circles or squares from your fabric, ensuring they are of the same size. Sew them together along the edges, leaving a small gap for stuffing. Fill the cushion with your chosen stuffing material until it reaches your preferred thickness. Then, sew the gap closed.

5. Ambient Lighting:

Soft lighting can create a serene atmosphere.

- Materials: Fairy lights, mason jars or lanterns.
- Instructions: Gently place the fairy lights inside the mason jars or lanterns. The result is a soft, glowing light source that can be placed around your meditation space.

By investing time in creating your meditation oasis, you infuse the space with personal energy and intention. Over time, this dedicated space becomes charged with meditative vibrations, helping you delve deeper into your practice.

Though don't feel restricted to the home. Some have found meditative comfort in other spaces. For many, nature offers the perfect backdrop for meditation. The gentle rustle of leaves, the rhythmic sound of waves crashing on a secluded beach, or the serene ambiance of a forest clearing can provide a profound sense of connection and grounding. In such places, the natural world's gentle hum enhances meditation, bringing a sense of oneness with the universe.

Cultural and Spiritual sites, Temples, churches, mosques, and other places of worship often radiate tranquility. Their spiritual significance and the collective energy of countless prayers and meditations can create a potent atmosphere for introspection. Even non-religious individuals can benefit from the serene ambiance these places often provide.

Community Centers and Dedicated Spaces in many cities offer meditation centers or community spaces with quiet rooms specifically designed for meditation and reflection. These spaces, often insulated from the city's noise and chaos, provide a communal sense of purpose, where collective energy can amplify the meditation experience.

Choosing a quiet place for meditation is akin to laying a strong foundation for a building. In silence, we minimize external distractions, allowing us to tune into our innermost thoughts and sensations more easily. The stillness amplifies our awareness, making it easier to observe our mind's patterns, let go of stress, and sink into a state of deep relaxation. In essence, a quiet environment acts as a catalyst, facilitating a more profound, more immersive meditative experience.

Body Position

Generally, when we talk about meditation, the most recommended body position for meditation is the seated posture, either on a cushion on the floor or in a chair. The spine should be upright, maintaining its natural curve, with the head balanced comfortably atop the neck. The hands can rest on the lap or the knees, and the eyes can be closed or kept slightly open, gazing downward. This posture promotes alertness, allows for proper breathing, and minimizes physical distractions, facilitating deeper meditation.

However, since our goal is to drift off to sleep, a different approach is recommended. Instead, a meditative lying down position, often referred to as the "Savasana" or "Corpse Pose" in yoga, is optimal for sleep meditation as it allows the practitioner to be fully supported and relaxed, facilitating a smooth transition from a state of mindful awareness to restful sleep.

When lying down for meditation, it's crucial to maintain a position that promotes relaxation, and physical comfort. Here are some essential points to keep in mind.

Surface Selection: Begin by choosing a comfortable and supportive surface, typically a bed or a yoga mat. If using a yoga mat, you might consider placing a soft blanket over it for added comfort.

Spinal Alignment: Ensure that your spine is straight and aligned, minimizing any curvature or twisting. This aids in free-flowing energy and unobstructed breathing. Lay on your back with your spine in its natural curve. This often means there's a small space between your lower back and the surface, which is perfectly fine. If there's an arch in your lower back and it's causing discomfort, consider placing a cushion or rolled-up towel or a folded blanket beneath your knees to reduce any strain.

Head Position: Your head should rest in a neutral position, aligned with your spine. Avoid tilting your chin too high or tucking it too closely to your chest. Using a flat pillow or a folded blanket can provide the right support without tilting the head excessively. Lay your head flat on the surface without using a high or stiff pillow.

If needed, use a thin pillow or a folded blanket to provide gentle support to the neck, ensuring that your neck aligns with the spine.

Awareness of Pressure Points: While lying down, be mindful of any areas that feel pressure or discomfort. These can be alleviated by adjusting your position slightly or using supportive props like cushions.

Breathing Space: Ensure your chest and abdomen are unrestricted, allowing for deep, natural breathing. Loose-fitting clothing can be helpful. As you settle into this position, take a few deep breaths, expanding your diaphragm and filling your lungs completely before exhaling slowly. Once you establish a rhythm, allow your breath to return to its natural flow.

Relaxed Limbs: Your arms and legs should be positioned in a manner that they're relaxed and free from strain. Avoid crossing your legs or having your arms in a tight or uncomfortable position.

Legs and Feet: Spread your legs hip-width apart, or slightly wider, allowing your feet to splay outwards naturally. This position avoids placing strain on the hips and ensures better blood circulation.

Arms and Hands: Rest your arms alongside your body but slightly apart, ensuring they don’t touch the sides of your body. This provides ample space for the lungs to expand freely during deep breathing. Your palms can face upwards, receptive to the energy around you, or downwards if that feels more grounding.

Facial Relaxation: It's common to hold tension in the face. Close your eyes gently, without pressing them shut. Soften your forehead, unclench your jaw, and part your teeth slightly, ensuring that your facial muscles are relaxed. Periodically check in and relax your forehead, eyebrows, eyes, and jaw. Softly parting your lips can help release tension in the jaw. Some people like to place a weighted eye mask or a soft cloth over their eyes for added relaxation.

Temperature Sensitivity: When lying still, you might feel colder over time. Ensure you're adequately covered or in a warm environment to avoid the distraction of feeling too cold.

Final Touches: Before immersing yourself in the meditation, do a quick scan from head to toe, releasing any tension you might find. This could be in your shoulders, your abdomen, or even in the soles of your feet.

Summary

Preparation is the cornerstone of a fruitful deep sleep meditation experience. It begins with a heartfelt commitment, signaling to oneself the sacredness of the practice and ensuring mental presence throughout the session. The importance of environment cannot be overstated; finding a serene, quiet spot, perhaps a dedicated corner of one's bedroom or a peaceful nook, becomes essential. In this undisturbed space, the external world fades, allowing for deeper introspection. Complementing this, adopting the right meditation position, particularly a comfortable lying down posture, bridges the gap between alert consciousness and restful slumber. With spine aligned, head comfortably rested, and limbs relaxed, the stage is set for a transformative journey into the realm of restful meditation.

5

One Powerful Guided Sleep Meditation

Hello, and welcome to this unique self-care session of guided meditation with mindfulness practices to lead you into a refreshing, more restorative deeper sleep.

Sleep, as we know, is vital for our overall well-being. Yet, in our modern, fast-paced world, achieving deep, restful sleep can sometimes be a challenge. So in this session we'll combine the art of meditation with the power of mindfulness, to help you find that inner tranquility.

Let's take a deep, cleansing breath together. In and out.

Commitment

Wherever you are in your sleep journey, regardless of whatever's going on in your life, take this moment to make a commitment to dedicate this time solely for your well-being.

Breath.

Together: "I commit this time to dedicate solely for my well-being."

Breath it in. Ah. Feel good?

Maybe you're a caregiver, a parent, or have responsibilities for someone else, even a pet. Maybe you're a provider and have work responsibilities. Regardless, this time is just for you.

Breath.

We're making a commitment right now to self-care, and to take time for ourselves to rest easy and drift off to sleep, letting go of all responsibilities.

And breath.

Maybe you've been struggling with sleep for a while now. Let's make a conscious choice to let go of the past. Release yesterday. Let it go and focus on the now.

Breath in.

Breath out.

Now.

Now is all there is.

A Quiet Place

If you haven't already, find a quiet place, a sanctuary where you can be undisturbed for the duration of this session. This could be your bedroom, a cozy corner, or any space where you feel safe and at ease.

Breath.

Take a moment to be grateful for this quiet space. Appreciate what feels good, what feels comfortable and easy about this space.

Breath.

Body Position

Now that you've found your quiet place, let's focus on the position of your body.

If you're sitting, plant your feet flat on the ground and feel the grounding energy of the earth beneath you.

If you're laying down, allow your body to fully relax into the support beneath you, feeling the stable presence of the earth cradling your form, grounding you in this moment of tranquility.

Feel free to gently shift your position and make any adjustments, much like a pet circles to find the perfect spot, until you settle into a position that's comfortable to you.

As we enter this meditation, allow yourself to make any small adjustments just like a cat settling into a cozy nook, seeking that perfect spot.

Getting Relaxed

Now we'll do a few exercises to help our bodies get relaxed.

Begin by softly pressing your lips together. As you exhale, part them slightly letting out a series of gentle, fluttering lip-trills. Repeat this thrice, feeling the tension in your jaw and facial muscles dissipate with each resonant trill.

Now, extend your arms out in front of you, and as you gently stretch, imagine reaching towards warmth and comfort. Hold this stretch for a few moments, inviting flexibility into your muscles. Slowly bring your arms back, noticing the space you've created in your body.

Feel relaxation pouring over your entire body.

Next, let's focus on tensing and relaxing. Clench your hands into fists, tense the muscles in your arms, hold this tension, notice it, then with an exhale, release it. Feel your muscles soften. Do the same with your legs – tense them tightly, and then let go, as if you're sinking deeper into relaxation with each release.

Now, bring attention to your shoulders. Gently roll them backwards in a slow, deliberate circular motion. Feel the loosening of any stiffness, the subtle unwinding of tightness. Reverse the direction, rolling forward now, continuing to usher ease into every movement.

Finally, with your spine long, tilt your head to one side, stretching the neck muscles. Hold this tender stretch for a moment before you switch to the other side. Allow each transition to be smooth and gentle, nurturing the areas that hold tension.

With each of these exercises, you're inviting tranquility into your body. Take a few moments in silence to let the effects of the relaxation seep deeper into your muscles, your mind.

Good.

Breathing

Now that we're in our relaxed, melting into our quiet place, let's take a moment to focus on our breathing.

Place one hand on your abdomen and the other on your chest. Inhale deeply through your nose, directing the breath down to your belly. Feel your belly rise more than your chest.

Breath in. Breath out.

This deep breathing encourages maximum oxygen uptake, signaling the body to activate its natural relaxation response. Exhale slowly through your mouth, feeling the belly lower.

Breath in. Breath out.

Let yourself decompress, and find a sense of calm in this deep belly breathing, letting each breath deepen your state of relaxation.

Breath in. Breath out.

Good.

Now we'll move into our 4-7-8 Breathing Technique. Inhale quietly through your nose for 4 seconds. Hold this breath for 7 seconds. This retention helps build up carbon dioxide, enhancing the calming effect when you exhale for 8 seconds, releasing tension. The slow exhale mimics the breathing pattern of sleep, preparing your body for rest.

Breath in through your nose. Count: 1-2-3.4.

Hold. Count: 1-2-3-4-5-6-7.

Breath out. Count: 1-2-3-4-5-6-7-8.

Holding your breath in for a count of seven seconds allows your lungs to fully inflate, facilitating the transfer of oxygen into your bloodstream and promoting a greater saturation of oxygen in your body.

Breath in through your nose. Count: 1-2-3.4.

Hold. Count: 1-2-3-4-5-6-7.

Breath out. Count: 1-2-3-4-5-6-7-8.

Feel the peace of relaxation.

Breath in through your nose. Count: 1-2-3.4.

Hold. Count: 1-2-3-4-5-6-7.

Breath out. Count: 1-2-3-4-5-6-7-8.

And we'll repeat one more time.

Breath in through your nose. Count: 1-2-3.4.

Hold. Count: 1-2-3-4-5-6-7.

Breath out. Count: 1-2-3-4-5-6-7-8.

Good.

Now we'll do an alternate nostril breathing exercise. Using your thumb and ring finger, gently close your right nostril and inhale through the left. Close the left nostril, open the right, and exhale. Inhale again through the right nostril, switch, and exhale through the left. This practice balances the hemispheres of the brain and calms the nervous system, preparing your body for rest.

Again, gently close the right nostril, and breath in.

And close the left nostril and breath in.

And for our last breathing exercise I want you to visualize a box as you breathe in for a count of four, hold for four, exhale for four, and hold again for four. This technique called "box breathing" helps to regulate the breathing pattern and can reduce stress, bringing a tranquil rhythm to your breath — a rhythm that invites sleep.

Breath in visualizing a box. Count 1-2-3-4.

Hold. Count: 1-2-3-4.

Exhale. Count: 1-2-3-4.

And Hold. Count: 1-2-3-4.

Good.

Take a deep breath in and breathe naturally, allowing the benefits of the exercises to permeate through your body.

By enhancing the oxygen supply to your body through these exercises, you help to improve circulation and reduce stress levels, both of which are conducive to better sleep. The deep, rhythmic breathing also helps to slow down your heartbeat, relax your muscles, and quiet your mind, setting the stage for restorative sleep.

Through breathing deeply, we increase the oxygen flow to our bloodstream, which can have a soothing effect on the body, decreasing stress hormones and helping the body transition into a state conducive to sleep.

With each exhale, feel yourself sinking deeper into the mattress, your muscles loosening, and your thoughts calming.

Guided Imagery

Close your eyes, and we'll do some visualization enhancing our sleep meditation journey with serene imagery to guide you even deeper into a peaceful slumber.

Imagine above you, a sky of the softest blue, dotted with fluffy, white clouds drifting lazily by. Each cloud morphs gently, taking the shape of your stresses and worries and carrying them away, leaving your mind clear and calm. With every breath, feel yourself lighter, as if you're floating among them, the sun's warm rays gently caressing your skin.

Now, picture a brilliant sunset on the horizon, its colors a vibrant tapestry of pinks, oranges, and purples. As the sun dips lower, it's as if all the day's energy is being reset, preparing you for the night. The colors soothe your mind, the fading light signaling to your body that it's time to rest.

Visualize yourself in a lush field of green grass, sprinkled with wildflowers nodding in a gentle breeze. The fragrance is calming, the soft buzz of nature's life a symphony for relaxation. You walk barefoot, the touch of the cool blades on your skin grounding you in this moment of peace.

As you continue this journey, see in your mind's eye the quiet beauty of autumn leaves falling gracefully to the ground. Each leaf represents a thought or a tension you're releasing, fluttering away, leaving space for stillness within you.

Now, imagine the flickering flame of a candle in a dimly lit room. The soft light casts a warm glow, the gentle dance of the flame hypnotic, inviting your mind to focus solely on its silent movement, everything else fading into the background.

Hear the soothing sounds of the ocean, waves rolling onto the shore in a steady, rhythmic pattern. With each wave, feel the embrace of tranquility. The waves moving with your breath.

Breath in.

Breath out.

Sense the tranquil murmur of water flowing over the soft mounds of sand on the beach, a natural lullaby for your soul.

And there, at the end of the shore, see a vibrant rainbow arching across the sky, a symbol of hope and peace, its colors bright against the clear, calming blue.

Envision a soft puppy, kitten or favorite pet asleep, its breaths even and serene. The innocence and trust in its restful slumber inspire you to let go of vigilance, to trust that each breath is a step closer to your own restful sleep.

Breath.

For a moment if you will go back to a memory of the last best sleep you can remember. Perhaps it was after a long run or bike ride; maybe the first time you got to sleep after finishing a big project, maybe it was after a night of passionate love making with someone very special to you and then you both fell fast asleep. There was a time after a really good meal, after a good day staying up late talking or out dancing with loved ones after which you fell in to bed and slept soundly for hours. How did that feel?

Breath.

Envision for yourself the best sleep ever. Maybe it was after the birth of your first child, if you're a parent; or perhaps a night when she or he started sleeping through the night. Maybe it was sometime in your own youth when you spent the whole day playing, carefree, or a time when you fell asleep in the warm embrace of a parent. Perhaps you were rocked to sleep in warm arms by someone who loves you and keeps you safe.

Now visualize take a moment to visualize your ideal sleeping place. Where are you? Maybe somewhere you took a lovely vacation. What's the air like? Gentle soft breezes. How does your body feel? Relaxed. Melting into a cozy bed. Warm under soft covers. See yourself in your ideal sleeping place dozing off, your eyes getting heavy as good sleep descends.

Allow these images to fill you with a sense of happiness and peace, washing over you wave by wave, breath by breath. And when you're ready, let these scenes slowly fade into the quiet darkness behind your closed eyes, leaving behind their essence, a residue of tranquility that lulls you into a deep, restorative sleep.

Breath.

Body Scan

Let's do a quick check-in, or body scan. Body scanning is a foundational practice in mindfulness, inviting a focused and nonjudgmental awareness to each part of the body in turn, promoting a state of deep relaxation and mental clarity.

Begin by bringing your attention to the very top of your head. Notice any sensations there, without judgment or expectation. With each exhale, imagine a wave of relaxation spreading from the top of your head down over your body. Let this sensation of calm wash over you, smoothing out the creases of your mind.

Now, shift your focus to your forehead. Smooth out any furrows, and let go of any tension with a long exhale. Move down to your eyes. Allow your eyelids to become heavy, feeling the tiny muscles around your eyes release and relax. Notice how this brings a deeper level of calm to your entire being.

Let this peaceful feeling flow over your cheeks and jaw, inviting these muscles to slacken. If your teeth are clenched, part them slightly, unburdening yourself of any lingering resistance.

Gently guide your awareness to your neck and shoulders. Encourage these areas to soften. Lift the weight of the world off your shoulders with each breath out, sinking further into relaxation.

Now, take your attention to your arms. Feel any sensations as you mentally trace down from your shoulders to your fingertips.

With each breath, release any holding, any tension, as you allow your arms to feel heavy and at ease.

Breathe into your chest and heart space, feeling the rise and fall with each breath. Send gratitude to your heart for its unwavering rhythm, and with an exhale, allow any emotional weight to dissolve.

As you scan down to your abdomen, honor the work your digestive system does for you. With your next out-breath, soften any tightness in this area.

Move your awareness to your back. Gently note any areas of tightness or discomfort and consciously relax these regions with each exhale. Allow the support of your bed to carry any burdens you've been holding onto.

Your attention now flows to your hips and pelvis, areas that may carry emotional stress. Inhale deeply, then exhale, imagining any stored tension melting away into the mattress.

Scan through your legs, from your thighs down to your feet. Acknowledge any sensations, and with kindness, encourage each muscle to soften, to release, with each out-breath. Feel your legs becoming heavy and relaxed.

Lastly, bring your attention to your feet. Release any remaining tension with one final, deep exhale, feeling your feet heavy and completely relaxed.

Now, with your entire body relaxed and your mind at ease, give yourself permission to drift into sleep. Let the natural rhythm of your breath guide you deeper into stillness, into rest, into peace. If your mind wanders, gently bring your focus back to your breath and the sensation of each body part sinking into relaxation.

Stay in this serene state, allowing sleep to come gently and naturally. When you awaken, may you feel refreshed and revitalized.

Use this body scan as a tool to bring about a state of deep relaxation, preparing you for a restful night's sleep. Allow the process to be gentle and natural, and remember that it's okay if you fall asleep during the meditation; it's a sign that it's working.

Clear your mind.

Clearing your mind is a central aspect of mindful meditation, essential for transitioning from the tumult of daily life into the non-physical realm of inner peace that promotes restful sleep. As you feel the air fill your lungs, and then slowly exhale, envisioning any stress or tension dissolving away.

Awareness of Thoughts

Acknowledge the thoughts crowding your mind—each one vying for attention—and then, with kindness, grant them permission to leave, making space for stillness. This clearing is the first step towards achieving a state where the non-physical essence of your consciousness can float free, unanchored from the worries of the waking world.

Imagine your thoughts as wisps of smoke that disperse and fade into nothingness with each out-breath. With each inhalation, draw in serenity; with each exhalation, release a day's worth of thoughts, commitments, and plans. As the boundaries of your mind expand, let the quiet envelop you, guiding you into the first stages of a peaceful, restorative meditation tailored for sleep.

As you clear your mind bring your attention to the present moment. Acknowledge that thoughts will arise. This is the mind's nature—to think. Mindfulness isn't about silencing your thoughts completely; it's about becoming aware of them.

Visualize your thoughts as leaves floating down a stream. They come into view, drift by, and disappear out of sight. Observe each one without attaching to it or pushing it away. If a thought demands attention, acknowledge it and then gently place it on a leaf, letting it float away. This is the essence of awareness—simply observing the ebb and flow of your mental landscape without getting swept away.

When the Mind Wanders

It's natural for the mind to wander. Sometimes, thoughts can pull you into the past or project you into the future. When you notice this happening, it's an opportunity to practice mindfulness. Observe where your mind has wandered without judgment. Each time you catch your mind drifting, it is a moment of mindfulness.

Gently guide your attention back to your breath, to the sensation of air entering and leaving your body, or to the ambient sounds that surround you. This act of returning your focus is like a mental muscle that gets stronger with practice. The wandering mind is not a failure but a chance to deepen your mindfulness.

Breath and be in the moment of this stillness, emptying your mind if only for a moment.

Centering Thoughts

Now center your thoughts. Imagine a space of stillness within you, like the eye of a storm where everything is calm and stable. Each time you breathe out, let this space expand, pushing out overactive thoughts and creating room for peace.

You can also use a word or phrase to bring your thoughts back to center. A mantra such as "peace" or "let go" on each exhale can be your anchor, drawing you back to a state of calm. Picture your mind as a sky, your thoughts as clouds, and your mantra helping to clear the sky, bringing it back to a state of serene blue openness.

The practice of clearing your mind is not about achieving a state of emptiness, but more about cultivating an environment where thoughts do not consume or define you. With mindfulness, you learn to coexist with your thoughts, to recognize them without being overwhelmed, and to maintain a gentle focus that keeps you anchored in the present moment.

Remember, the goal of mindfulness is not to battle with your thoughts, but to build an awareness that helps you recognize and appreciate the space between them. It's in this space that clarity and tranquility reside.

As the final minutes of our meditation unfold, it's time to seamlessly transition from a state of mindful awareness to the welcoming arms of sleep. Allow the cadence of your breath to become your lullaby, guiding you toward slumber. With each inhale, draw in peace; with each exhale, let go of the day. Feel your body sinking deeper into relaxation, every muscle unwinding, every tension unraveling.

Breath in. Breath out.

Conclude Gracefully

As this meditation comes to an end imagine yourself as a leaf carried softly by a gentle stream, floating effortlessly toward a vast, tranquil ocean of rest. The boundaries between wakefulness and dream begin to blur as you drift on the edge of consciousness. This is your journey from the physical to the ethereal, from the known to the mysterious embrace of the night.

As you let go, your breaths become softer, your awareness of the external world dims, and the soothing darkness behind your closed eyelids invites you in. There's nothing to do now but surrender to the quiet promise of sleep, allowing it to enfold you in its velvet tapestry.

You might no longer be consciously hearing my words, as you're at the threshold of sleep, where the mind rests and rejuvenates. Embrace this natural progression from meditation to sleep, where every gentle breath draws you closer to sweet dreams.

Let this graceful conclusion to your meditation be a silent vow that you carry within—a commitment to allow healing rest to come as it will, knowing you are safe, you are at peace, and you are surrounded by the gentle tranquility.

And now, sleep awaits. There's nowhere else you need to be, nothing else you need to do. Allow yourself to drift off, carried by the waves of your own calm breathing, to wherever you may be lying. Goodnight, and may you have a restful journey into sleep.

6

Music For Self-Reflection

If you're listening to the audio version, you'll hear gentle music for self-reflection with 528 Hz binaural beats as a sleep aid.

7

Introduction To White Noise

The granular static noise characteristic of white noise has been known to enhance sleep for many. It operates by drowning out ambient sounds. A recent study revealed that white noise expedited sleep onset for 38% of participants.[1]

This research looks at the relationship between white noise and sleep quality. The scientific rationale behind this is related to how our brain processes sounds. In the presence of a consistent sound like white noise, the brain tends to relax, reducing the time it takes to transition from full wakefulness to sleep.

White noise has long been championed as an aid to induce sleep, and its unique properties offer several advantages for those seeking a restful night. At its core, white noise is a consistent sound that contains equal intensities of all frequencies audible to the human ear. This consistent sonic backdrop offers numerous benefits to sleep quality, with science validating its effectiveness.

---

[1] "White Noise, Pink Noise, and Brown Noise: What's the Difference?" Medically Reviewed by Melinda Ratini, MS, DO on July 12, 2022 Written by Kara Mayer Robinson, WebMD, https://www.webmd.com/sleep-disorders/pink-noise-sleep

One of the primary advantages of white noise is its ability to drown out mask ambient sounds. Whether it's the honk of a car, the chirping of early morning birds, or the hum of an air conditioner, these sporadic noises can disrupt our sleep. By providing a constant auditory backdrop, white noise effectively masks these disturbances, ensuring that sudden changes in the acoustic environment are less noticeable and, therefore, less disruptive.

The consistent nature of white noise can also have a calming effect on the brain. It promotes relaxation. Just as the repetitive sound of rain or the rhythm of waves crashing can be soothing, the even tones of white noise can help lull the brain into a state of relaxation, paving the way for sleep.

For some, Deep sleep, REM sleep, and the transitional phases in between can all be vulnerable to acoustic disruptions. White noise, by offering a steady auditory experience, a consistency across sleep cycles that ensures that even as we cycle through these stages of sleep, we remain shielded from potential disturbances, fostering a deeper and more restful night.

Overall, white noise acts as a sonic guardian, protecting our sleep from the unpredictable sounds of the environment. Its consistent, soothing nature not only masks disturbances but also beckons the brain into a tranquil state conducive to sleep, as supported by scientific studies. For many, it's a simple yet profound tool in the quest for a good night's rest.

8

White Noise Meditation

Welcome to this white noise meditation. One of the most challenging and at the same time most powerful things you can do in meditation is to clear your mind. Take a moment and let the sound of white noise fill your space.

Think of this steady auditory backdrop as an invisible eraser. As thoughts come in, allow the mist of white noise to gently wipe them away.

In this mediation we are making a commitment to use this time to clear our minds.

If you haven't already, find a quite space where you feel comfortable and at ease.

Get into a comfortable position either sitting or lying down. Align your spine. If you're sitting imagine a string pulling your spine up straight to the sky. If you're laying down, align your spine horizontally.

Breath 1-2-3-4, and relax.

And again 1-2-3-4, and relax.

Let's do a few exercises for a deeper relaxation of the body with a squeeze and then release, starting from our toes.

Start with the right leg. Curl your toes, squeezing them together. Curl your foot, arching it to get that stretch. Breath and release.

We'll squeeze our lower left leg, stretching our ankle and tightening our calf. Breath and release.

We'll tighten our upper leg and thigh all the way up to the buttocks and squeeze. Breath and release.

Now the left leg. Starting with our toes again squeeze them together, and arch your foot feeling that stretch all the way into the ankle. Breath and release.

Continuing with the left leg, let's focus on the lower leg. Engage the muscles in your lower left leg, feeling the stretch in your ankle and the tightening in your calf. Take a deep breath in, hold it for a moment, and as you breathe out, release the tension. Feel the relaxation spreading through your lower leg.

Now, move to your upper left leg. Tighten the muscles in your thigh, all the way up to your buttocks. Squeeze these muscles gently, feeling the engagement throughout your upper leg. Take another deep breath, and as you exhale, gradually release the tension. Allow a sense of calm to wash over your upper leg.

Shifting focus to the stomach or core area, start by taking a deep breath in. As you inhale, tighten your abdominal muscles, pulling your navel towards your spine. Hold this tension briefly, feeling the core muscles engage and strengthen. Then, as you exhale, slowly relax your abdominal muscles. Feel the release of tension across your stomach, allowing your breath to flow naturally and your body to sink into deeper relaxation.

This sequence of tensing and relaxing muscles, starting from the right leg and moving up to the core, not only helps in relaxation but also enhances body awareness and mindfulness.

Now let's focus on our chest and upper back. Start by sitting or standing with a straight spine. Inhale deeply and, as you do, expand your chest outward, pulling your shoulder blades slightly towards each other. This movement engages the muscles in your upper back and chest. Hold this expanded, open position for a few seconds, feeling the stretch and tension across your chest and the contraction in your upper back. Then, as you exhale, gently release the tension, allowing your chest to return to its natural position.

Now, focus on the middle and lower parts of your back. Take another deep breath, and as you inhale, arch your back slightly, engaging the muscles in your middle and lower back. Be gentle and avoid straining; the movement should be comfortable and smooth. Hold this arch for a moment, feeling the stretch and engagement of the back muscles. Then, on the exhale, gently release the arch, allowing your spine to return to a neutral, relaxed position.

Then we'll bring our attention to our shoulders and neck. Inhale deeply, and as you do, lift your shoulders towards your ears, creating a slight tension in your shoulder and neck muscles. Hold this lifted position for a few seconds, then, as you exhale, gently roll your shoulders back and down, releasing any tension. Feel the relaxation spread from your shoulders up through your neck.

Now let's focus on our arms for a bit, starting with the right arm. Inhale deeply, and as you do, make a fist with your right hand, squeezing your fingers tightly. Extend this tension up your right arm, engaging the muscles in your forearm, elbow, and upper arm.

Feel the strength and tension all the way from your fingers to your shoulder. Hold this for a few seconds, then, as you exhale, gradually release the tension, starting from your fingers, unfolding them slowly, and then relaxing your arm muscles. Feel the wave of relaxation travel from your fingertips up to your shoulder.

Now, shift your focus to your left arm. Inhale deeply, and as you breathe in, folding your left hand into a fist, squeezing your fingers together. Extend this tension through your left arm, engaging the muscles in your forearm, around your elbow, and into your upper arm. Notice the sensation of strength and tightness along your entire arm. Hold this position for a moment, and then, as you exhale, begin to relax your hand, unfurling your fingers first, and then easing the tension in your forearm, elbow, and upper arm. Allow the relaxation to spread, releasing any tension held in your left arm.

Inhale deeply continuing up the spine to your neck. As you do, gently tilt your head back slightly, feeling a stretch in the front of your neck. Be careful not to strain. Hold this position for a few seconds, then slowly exhale and bring your head back to a neutral position.

Next, inhale and gently tilt your head forward, chin towards chest, to stretch the back of your neck. Hold briefly, then exhale and return to the neutral position. Repeat these movements gently, allowing the neck muscles to relax and release any tension.

Breath in then slowly exhale, gently washing away any thoughts, clearing your mind.

Now we'll shift our attention to our facial muscles. Inhale, and scrunch up your facial muscles. Squint your eyes, pucker your lips, wrinkle your nose. Hold this tension for a few seconds, 1-2-3-4, then, as you exhale, gradually release all the tension, smoothing out your facial expression. It's nice to stretch a little, opening your mouth, and a little yawn or verbal exhale is okay as you relax. Let's do it together, "Ah." Yes. Feel the relaxation spreading across your face.

Inhale and clench your jaw, feeling the tension in your cheeks and temples. Be careful not to overdo it to avoid discomfort. Hold this clench for a few seconds, then exhale and relax your jaw, letting your mouth fall slightly open and the muscles around your temples release. You might gently massage your temples in small circular motions to enhance relaxation.

Now let's consider our whole body as we inhale deeply, filling our lungs completely. Gradually start squeezing and tensing every muscle group in your body, starting from your feet, tensing your toes, feet, and calves.

Move up through your legs, squeezing your thigh muscles, then engage your buttocks, core, chest, back, and arms all the way down to your hands, making fists. Finally, gently clench your jaw and squeeze your eyes shut, tensing the facial muscles. Your entire body.

Hold this full-body tension for a few seconds. Feel the energy in every part of your body. Now, very gently begin to stretch, extending your arms and legs, reaching out as if you're trying to touch the opposite walls with your fingertips and toes. Extend your stretch as much as comfortably possible, elongating your body.

Breath in deeply 1-2-3-4. Now exhale slowly releasing the tension in every muscle group, beginning from your head and face, moving down through your neck, shoulders, arms, chest, back, core, hips, thighs, legs, and finally your feet. Feel each part of your body becoming heavier and more relaxed as you exhale. As you release all the tension, imagine your body sinking into a state of complete relaxation.

Continue to breathe deeply and rhythmically. With each inhale 1-2-3-4, imagine calmness and clarity entering your body. With each exhale, visualize stress and tension leaving your body. Imagine your mind clearing. Allow yourself a few moments in this state of deep relaxation and mental clarity. Feel your mind becoming more serene and your body completely relaxed.

This whole-body exercise not only helps in releasing physical tension but also aids in clearing your mind, fostering a sense of peace and rejuvenation. Perform these steps slowly and mindfully, paying attention to your body and breath, ensuring a harmonious connection between mind and body.

Feel the easiness of your entire body being relaxed. Breath into that feeling of comfort and ease, sinking into peace and tranquility.

Now we'll close our eyes and take a few deep, calming breaths to center ourselves. Inhale slowly and deeply through your nose, filling your lungs completely. Hold your breath for a moment 1-2-3-4, then exhale slowly and fully through your mouth. As you breathe, let go of any wandering thoughts, concerns or tension.

In this field of soothing white noise visualize a sky filled with clouds. These clouds represent your thoughts, worries, and daily distractions. See them in various shapes and sizes, moving slowly across your mental sky.

As you continue to breathe deeply, imagine that with each exhale, you're gently blowing the clouds away. With every breath out, more clouds disperse, slowly revealing glimpses of the clear, serene sky behind them.

Gradually, with each breath, the sky becomes clearer. The clouds thin out, revealing more of the bright, peaceful blue sky. Feel the sense of openness and calmness as the sky in your mind becomes completely clear. Enjoy the vastness and tranquility of this clear sky.

Whenever you find your thoughts trying to wander back in, refocus on the sound of the white noise. Let it fill the spaces where thoughts try to intrude, just like a gentle breeze that keeps the sky clear. Allow the consistent sound of the white noise to anchor your mind, helping you maintain the clear-sky visualization.

Deepening our focus on white noise, immerse yourself in the sound of the white noise, let it become the central focus of your awareness.

Now picture yourself sitting or standing on a beautiful, serene beach. The sand is soft and warm under your feet, and in front of you stretches the vast, calm ocean. The sky above is a clear blue, and the sun gently warms your skin. This beach is your mental sanctuary, a place of peace and tranquility.

As you focus on the white noise, imagine it transforming into the sound of gentle ocean waves. Each wave rolls in smoothly towards the shore, cresting softly before washing over the sand. These waves are rhythmic and steady, calming the entire beach with their gentle motion.

As these waves reach the shore, visualize them gently washing over any footprints in the sand – these footprints symbolize your worries, distractions, and intrusive thoughts. With each wave, the footprints become fainter and fainter, until they are completely gone, leaving the sand smooth and unmarked. Your mind mirrors this clarity, becoming more peaceful and serene with each passing wave.

Deepen the relaxation with each wave. Imagine that each sound wave from the white noise is like a gentle wave washing over a beach, smoothing out and clearing any footprints – these footprints that represent your intrusive thoughts. With each wave of sound, your mind becomes more serene, like a pristine, untouched beach.

With every wave that washes ashore, feel your body relax further. Let the rhythmic sound of the waves guide your breathing – inhale as the wave gathers strength, and exhale as it washes ashore, releasing tension and clearing your mind.

Let the easy tranquility of the white noise waves wash over you. Visualize the warmth of the sun, the softness of the sand, the vastness of the ocean, and the clearness of the sky. This beach is a safe space for you, always available whenever you need to escape from the chaos of everyday life.

Allow the imagery of the clear sky to merge with the sound of white noise. Visualize that the sound is not only keeping the sky clear, but also adding to its tranquility. The white noise becomes a part of the peaceful sky, filling the expanse with a soft, soothing texture. It's as if the clear sky and the white noise are harmoniously intertwined, creating a space of profound peace and clarity.

Breath in 1-2-3-4, breath out. Align your breathing with the rhythm of the white noise. Inhale slowly and deeply as the sound seems to rise, and exhale gently as the sound naturally fades. This synchronization helps in deepening the relaxation and enhancing mental clarity. Feel your breath and the white noise becoming one – a symphony of calmness.

As thoughts come in, gently acknowledge them without judgment and imagine them being encapsulated in soft, white clouds.

As you focus back on the white noise, visualize these clouds being gently blown away, leaving behind only the clear, calm sky and the harmonious sound of the white noise.

As you immerse yourself in this white noise and the visualization, it's natural for thoughts to emerge. These could be about your day, plans, worries, or random memories. When a thought arises, the first step is to recognize its presence. Instead of trying to force it away or feeling frustrated, simply acknowledge that the thought has appeared.

We're going to apply something called, "Non-Judgmental Observation." Approach these thoughts with a stance of non-judgment and curiosity. Imagine if you will that you are just an impartial observer, watching these thoughts float by. There's no need to label them as good or bad, or to engage with their content. Just notice them – "Here is a thought about work," or "Here is a memory." This practice helps in detaching from the thought and reduces its impact.

Here we are visualizing our thoughts as objects, nothing to worry or distract us from clearing our minds. Visualize each thought as a physical object, like a leaf floating down a stream or a cloud passing in the sky. The white noise in the background can serve as the gentle current of the stream or the breeze moving the clouds. As a thought appears, see it settling on a leaf or cloud, and then gently being carried away by the natural flow of the sound waves.

As you listen to the white noise, visualizing a peaceful, gentle stream filled will clear, fresh water in a serene natural setting. This stream flows smoothly and effortlessly, surrounded by lush greenery and bathed in soft, warm sunlight.

In your mind's eye, see a single leaf gently falling from a tree and landing on the surface of the stream. This leaf is light and floats easily. It represents your thoughts, emotions, or any distractions that might arise during your meditation.

As thoughts or distractions enter your mind, visualize them settling onto the leaf. Maybe it's a worry, a plan, or just a random thought. Place each thought on the leaf and watch as the current of the stream of white noise just carries the leaf away.

Notice how the leaf with your thought on it floats downstream, moving away from you. It doesn't sink or struggle; it simply drifts along with the flow of the water. This represents the natural flow and impermanence of thoughts – they come, but they also go.

Each time a thought is placed on a leaf and sent downstream, bring your focus back to the flowing water, allowing the white noise to clear your mind. This represents the present moment – constant, continuous, and always available to you.

After acknowledging and visualizing the thought drifting away, gently redirect your focus back to the white noise. Let the consistent, soothing sound guide you back to a state of calm focus. The white noise serves as a reminder to return to the present moment, offering a sound-based anchor for your attention.

Each time you successfully acknowledge a thought and return to your focus on the white noise, you deepen your state of relaxation and mindfulness. This practice reinforces your ability to handle distractions and enhances your overall meditation experience.

Regular practice of acknowledging thoughts without judgment during white noise meditation can improve your ability to maintain focus and tranquility in everyday life. This expanded approach to dealing with intrusive thoughts during white noise meditation is a key aspect of mindfulness practice. It encourages a healthier relationship with your thoughts, fostering a sense of peace and clarity in your mental landscape.

Spend a few minutes enjoying the serene peacefulness of your visualization. Stay in this peaceful state as long as you need. When you feel fully relaxed and your mind feels clear, slowly start to bring your awareness back to your physical surroundings. Take a moment to appreciate the calmness and clarity you've cultivated. Gently wiggle your fingers and toes, take a deep breath, and when you're ready, open your eyes.

9

White Noise Recording

If you're listening to the audio version, you'll hear a segment of white noise with 528 Hz binaural beats for better sleep.

10

Introduction To Gratitude Meditation

Some of you might be wondering, "Why is there a gratitude meditation in a book about better sleep?" Well, one thing that people often don't connect with better sleep, but that can really have a profound effect on sleep quality, is gratitude. It turns out that incorporating gratitude into your meditation practice has a uniquely positive impact on sleep, offering various psychological and physiological benefits that contribute to improved sleep quality.

One of the most significant effects of gratitude on sleep is its ability to reduce stress and anxiety. Grateful people tend to ruminate less on negative thoughts, which are often a source of nighttime anxiety and sleep disturbances. By focusing on positive aspects of life and acknowledging the good, gratitude shifts attention away from stressors and worries that can hinder the onset and quality of sleep. This shift in focus promotes a more relaxed state of mind, making it easier to fall asleep.

The effect of gratitude on sleep is supported by various studies and research findings. Gratitude has been shown to predict greater subjective sleep quality and sleep duration, and less sleep latency and daytime dysfunction. This relationship is mediated by more positive pre-sleep cognitions and less negative pre-sleep cognitions, as indicated in a study published on PubMed.[2]

Additionally, practicing gratitude can help manage negative emotions like guilt and shame, which are often linked to stress, depression, and anxiety. By reducing these negative emotions, gratitude indirectly improves sleep quality. Keeping a gratitude journal or consistently verbalizing gratitude has been suggested as effective methods for managing these emotions and enhancing physical health.[3]

Furthermore, gratitude's role in lowering stress hormones and offering a positive perspective is crucial for promoting better sleep, ultimately aiding in the management of emotional well-being. This approach helps in alleviating anxiety, a common barrier to restful sleep.[4]

These findings collectively highlight how gratitude, through its positive impact on emotional and mental health, can significantly improve sleep quality and duration. The practice of gratitude, whether through journaling or other means, serves as a valuable tool in fostering a healthier sleep cycle.

Gratitude is closely linked with an increase in positive emotions like happiness, contentment, and optimism. These positive

---

[2] "Gratitude influences sleep through the mechanism of pre-sleep cognitions." PubMed. Available at: https://pubmed.ncbi.nlm.nih.gov/19073292/.

[3] "Practicing Gratitude for Better Health and Well-Being." University of Utah Health. Available at: https://healthcare.utah.edu/healthfeed/2021/11/practicing-gratitude-better-health-and-well-being.

[4] "Gratitude and Anxiety: The Natural Road to Improved Mental Health." Well.org. Available at: https://well.org/mindset/gratitude-and-anxiety-all-natural-road-improved-mental-health.

emotional states are conducive to a more peaceful mind at bedtime. People who regularly practice gratitude are more likely to go to bed with positive thoughts, which can lead to a more restful and undisturbed sleep. Positive emotions have been shown to facilitate the rapid onset of sleep and reduce the occurrence of wakefulness during the night.

Regular expressions of gratitude can actually improve the overall quality of sleep. Studies have shown that gratitude is associated with better sleep quality, longer sleep duration, and less difficulty falling asleep. This improvement is partly due to the calming effect gratitude has on the mind, but it also relates to the overall healthier lifestyle choices that often accompany a grateful mindset, such as exercising more and engaging in healthier social interactions.

Incorporating gratitude into a nightly routine can create a calming bedtime ritual. Reflecting on positive aspects of the day, or even mentally acknowledging things to be grateful for can establish a habit of relaxation and positivity before sleep. This practice helps in winding down and prepares the mind and body for rest.

Gratitude can be an effective tool against the negative thought patterns often seen in insomnia. By intentionally acknowledging the positive aspects of life, individuals can redirect their focus away from the racing, often negative thoughts that can accompany sleeplessness. This cognitive shift can reduce the time it takes to fall asleep and can improve the overall sleep experience.

Incorporating gratitude into sleep meditation can significantly enhance the depth and quality of sleep, benefiting both mental and physical health. By replacing worrisome or anxious thoughts with gratitude, the mind settles into a more peaceful state, conducive to deeper sleep. This shift in mindset not only helps in falling asleep faster but also in achieving a more restful, uninterrupted sleep cycle.

Gratitude has been shown to lower levels of cortisol, the body's primary stress hormone. Engaging in gratitude practices, such as counting blessings and gratitude letter writing, can lead to about a 23% reduction in cortisol levels.[5] Elevated cortisol levels, especially at night, can disrupt the natural sleep-wake cycle and prevent deep sleep. By engaging in gratitude meditation, individuals can lower their stress response, allowing the body to enter a more relaxed state. This relaxation is crucial for transitioning into the deeper stages of sleep, such as slow-wave sleep (deep sleep) and REM sleep, which are vital for physical restoration and memory consolidation.[6]

Gratitude meditation can directly impact the quality of sleep by promoting more positive pre-sleep cognitions, as evidenced in various studies. A mindset of gratitude helps create a more optimistic and content state of mind, which is linked to better sleep quality. People who regularly engage in gratitude practices report fewer sleep disturbances and improved sleep quality.

The practice of gratitude has a strong connection with overall emotional health. By reflecting on positive aspects of life and expressing thankfulness, individuals can improve their mood and overall sense of well-being. This positive emotional state is not only beneficial for mental health but also for physical health, as it promotes

---

[5] "Gratitude is good medicine." UC Davis Health. Available at: https://health.ucdavis.edu/medicalcenter/features/2015-2016/11/20151125_gratitude.html.

[6] "How to Get More Deep Sleep: Maximizing Your Restorative Rest." Sleep Foundation. Available at: https://www.sleepfoundation.org/stages-of-sleep/how-to-get-more-deep-sleep.

relaxation and deeper sleep. A better emotional state at bedtime can enhance the body's ability to rejuvenate during sleep.

Incorporating gratitude into sleep meditation can become a relaxing bedtime ritual that signals the body it's time to wind down. This ritual can involve silently expressing thanks, or meditating on feelings of gratitude. Such rituals are effective in creating a calm and comforting bedtime environment, making it easier for the mind and body to prepare for deep sleep.

In summary, the practice of gratitude can play a significant role in enhancing sleep quality. Its ability to foster positive emotions, reduce stress and anxiety, and establish relaxing bedtime routines contributes to better sleep hygiene and overall well being. Given these benefits, incorporating gratitude into daily life may be a simple yet powerful way to improve both mental health and sleep. Incorporating gratitude into sleep meditation can lead to deeper, more restorative sleep by fostering a positive mindset, reducing stress levels, and improving overall emotional well-being. This practice, as part of a regular bedtime routine, can significantly enhance sleep quality and contribute to better overall health.

11

Gratitude Sleep Meditation

Welcome to your gratitude sleep meditation. Embracing gratitude can profoundly enhance your vibrational energy, creating a pathway to realizing your aspirations. Engage in this gratitude meditation daily, and observe a remarkable transformation in your life. As you drift into a state of deeper, more restful sleep, let gratitude for your current blessings and future manifestations fill your heart. In this vast expanse of consciousness, your realization of better, deeper sleep awaits. Through gratitude, you draw aspects of quality sleep ever closer to your own experience, amplifying your ability to materialize them. This practice is not just a ritual; it's a powerful tool in shaping the life you dream of.

Now let's close our eyes and put everything else aside for a while to dedicate this time, this present moment, to focus on gratitude. If you haven't already, let's find a quite spot where you won't be distracted for a while. Get into a comfortable position - it could be a chair, meditation cushion, or laying down in your bed, wherever or however you feel comfortable and at ease. Align your spine so it's relatively straight. Take a deep breath in 1-2-3-4, and breath out.

Nice. Again in 1-2-3-4, and out. One more time: breath in 1-2-3-4, and out. Feel good?

While we may feel tired or even frustrated, there's alway something in our day, in our experience that we can be grateful for, no matter how small. When we think about it there are so many tiny things that may happen throughout our days that we may deem at the time as inconsequential, maybe not even have noticed. Maybe the sound of laughter, whether it's from loved ones or strangers, it's a universal sign of joy. Maybe home comforts like the warmth of a blanket or the familiarity of a favorite chair. Maybe there was a blooming flower on your way out the door, a clear blue sky, maybe a compliment or some small act of kindness someone made. Whatever it is, find it and take a moment to savor it and be thankful.

Let's start with being thankful for our bodies and all of their intricate working parts. The human body is truly amazing, and we are thankful. Let the universe know. Say: "Thank you for my body." And it's fine to say it in your head. Think about all the things in your body that have to go right just to move a finger. It's remarkable. The muscles in your finger have to receive a nerve signal all the way from neurons up in your brain - quite a journey. Blood vessels have to provide the right amount of oxygen for your finger muscles to contract. There has to be an adequate supply of synovial fluid and healthy cartilage for the joints in your knuckles to bend. It's a symphony. And we say what? "Thank you." There's so much to be grateful for.

And let's remember to breath in 1-2-3-4, and breath out. Breath in 1-2-3-4, and breath out, letting all the tension of the day leave our bodies.

Focus your attention on your lower body. Feel the weight of your hips, legs, and feet. Visualize roots growing from these areas, extending deep into the earth. This imagery helps create a sense of stability and grounding. As you breathe in, imagine drawing energy up from the earth. As you breathe out, envision any tension or restlessness flowing down into the ground. This process enhances your connection to the earth, providing a stable foundation that promotes calmness and prepares your body for restful sleep.

Feel the surface beneath you supporting your buttocks and lower back. Turning your attention to this area, notice any sensations here as you breathe in deeply and exhale slowly. With each exhale, imagine any tightness or discomfort in your buttocks and lower back melting away. Feel these areas becoming softer and more relaxed.

Picture a warm, comforting light enveloping your this area of your body, providing support and relief. Connect with the Earth, visualizing roots extending from your lower back and buttocks, grounding you deeply into the earth. With each inhale, draw up stability and calm from the earth.

Gently acknowledge and thank this part your body for its strength and support, for carrying you through the day. Allow yourself to sink deeper into relaxation, getting closer to a deep restorative sleep.

Focus your attention on your stomach and chest. Take deep breaths, feeling your stomach rise and fall, and your chest expand and contract. As you breathe out, let go of any tension in this area. Imagine stress and tightness dissolving with each exhale.

Softly roll your shoulders forward, back and down. Do this slowly a few times to release any held tension in the shoulder area. Picture a soothing wave of relaxation starting from your stomach, moving up through your chest, and flowing over your shoulders, carrying away stress and strain.

Acknowledge the work your stomach, chest, and shoulders do. Feel grateful for their strength and resilience. With each breath, feel more relaxed and serene, as your upper body sinks into a state of peacefulness, preparing you for restful sleep.

Bring your attention to your lower back, gradually moving up to your upper back. Feel the surface supporting these areas. Inhale deeply and, as you exhale, let go of any tension in your back. Visualize tightness in your muscles unwinding. Reverse Shoulder Roll: Slowly roll your shoulders backward this time, up, and then back down in a fluid motion. This helps release tension from the upper back and encourages alignment.

Imagine a wave of warmth and relaxation starting at your lower back and moving upward, smoothing and softening muscles as it ascends. Acknowledge the support your back provides daily. Feel grateful for its strength and flexibility. Now with each breath, sink deeper into relaxation. Breath in 1-2-3-4, and breath out. Yes. Breath in 1-2-3-4, and breath out. Feeling your back fully supported and at ease, readying you for a restful night's sleep.

Gently shift your focus to your arms and neck. Feel their weight and position. Breathe in deeply, and as you exhale, imagine tension flowing out of your arms and neck. Allow them to become more relaxed with each breath.

Now slowly lift your arms, stretch them out, and then gently lower them, encouraging blood flow and relaxation. Carefully tilt your head from side to side, easing any tightness in the neck muscles. Picture a soothing energy enveloping your arms and neck, easing any discomfort or stiffness.

Take a moment to appreciate your arms for their functionality and your neck for its support and flexibility. Continue to breathe deeply, feeling your arms and neck sinking into a relaxed state, preparing your body for a tranquil and restful sleep.

And finally bring your attention to your head and the area around your temples. Notice any sensations you may feel. Inhale slowly and deeply, then exhale gently, allowing any tension in your head and temples to dissipate.

Using your fingertips, softly massage your temples in a circular motion. This can help alleviate tension headaches and promote relaxation. Imagine a wave of calmness starting at the top of your head, washing over your temples, soothing and releasing any stress.

Take a moment to reflect on the vital functions your head and brain perform every day and feel thankful for them. As you continue with slow, deep breaths, feel your head and temples relax further, contributing to a state of tranquility, ideal for deep and restful sleep.

In gratitude we bring ourselves closer to inner peace and with that closer to better sleep. By shifting our focus from what we lack to what we have, we promote a positive mindset in ourselves, reduce stress, and enhance our overall sense of well-being. And by acknowledging and appreciating the good in our lives, we foster a sense of contentment and serenity for better sleep.

Now that our bodies are relaxed, appreciated, and ready for sleep, I'm going to kick off a little gratitude rampage, so to speak. I'll say something like, "I'm thankful for the sunset." And if it's also something that you're thankful for, or that resonates with you, just let it echo and reverberate in your consciousness. And if it's something that made you feel good, like a warm drink or a nice hug, we want to ruminate in it, and enjoy it. Okay. And feel free to add your own things you are thankful for in this welcome space of gratitude. Or amend or add your flavor on it. Like if I say, "I'm thankful for ice cream," for you maybe it's "chocolate ice cream" or I don't know, "raspberry ripple." Sound good? Okay.

Let's begin with gratitude for our physical well-being and comfort.

Thank you for my healthy body, allowing me to embrace life's adventures.

Thank you for my strong bones, providing the framework for my physical presence.

Thank you for my strong muscles, empowering me to move and engage with the world.

Thank you for my healthy heart, sustaining life with every pulse.

Thank you for my strong back, supporting me through each day's challenges and tasks.

Thank you for my legs, carrying me on my journey through life's paths.

Thank you for my feet, grounding me to the earth with every step.

Thank you for my arms, enabling me to hold my loved ones close and interact with the world.

Thank you for my hands, with which I create, express, and heal.

Thank you for my eyes, the lenses that bring the colors of the world into view.

Thank you for my ears, channeling the harmonies and messages of life.

Thank you for my taste buds, letting me enjoy the diversity of flavors life offers.

Thank you for my healthy digestive system, processing the nourishment I receive from food.

Thank you for my balanced nervous system, coordinating my body's actions and responses.

Thank you for my ability to communicate and share my thoughts and feelings with others.

Thank you for the agility and flexibility of my body, allowing me to move freely and with ease.

Thank you for the restorative power of sleep, which rejuvenates me every night.

Thank you for the breath in my lungs, a constant rhythm that sustains me without thought.

Thank you for the intricate balance of my inner systems working in harmony to keep me well.

Thank you for the sensation of touch, enabling me to experience the comfort of texture and warmth.

Thank you for the ability to rest and relax, essential for my physical and mental recovery.

Thank you for the natural healing processes of my body, mending and maintaining my well-being day by day.

Thank you for the nourishment I receive from food, which fuels my vitality and health.

Thank you for the resilience that surfaces in challenging times, reminding me of my inner strength.

Thank you for my capacity to learn from every situation, turning experiences into wisdom.

Thank you for the unique talents I possess, allowing me to contribute my creativity to the world.

Thank you for the joy I find in little moments, enriching my daily life with happiness.

Thank you for the confidence to stand up for what I believe in and to make my voice heard.

Thank you for the love I have the privilege to give and receive, creating meaningful connections.

Thank you for my curiosity that leads me to explore, discover, and grow beyond my boundaries.

Thank you for the laughter and playfulness that keep my spirit young and my heart light.

Take a breath. Ah. Again. Breath in. Breath out.

Now we'll take some time to give thanks for some of the daily essentials in our lives and in our homes.

Thank you for the sunrise that greets me each morning, a daily promise of a fresh start.

Thank you for the access to fresh produce, enriching my diet with nature's vitality.

Thank you for the peace of mind that comes with a secure living space, where I can rest and recharge.

Thank you for the convenience of modern plumbing, a luxury that makes cleanliness a simple part of life.

Thank you for the cozy bedding that cradles me each night, offering rest and comfort.

Thank you for the warmth of heating and the coolness of air conditioning, making my home a haven through the seasons.

Thank you for the means of communication that keep me informed and engaged in the tapestry of human knowledge and current events.

Thank you for the soothing presence of houseplants, bringing a touch of nature's calm into my personal space.

Thank you for my cozy kitchen, where the aroma of home-cooked meals fills the air and where I whipped up a perfect pasta dinner that brought smiles all around the table.

Thank you for my sunny breakfast nook, where my kids proudly make their own breakfast, filling the space with early morning giggles and a sense of growing independence.

Thank you for the perfectly sized window above my kitchen sink, offering me a view of my garden's blooming flowers, making even the simple act of sipping tea feel like a moment of serene connection with nature.

Thank you for my comfortable living room sofa, where countless family stories are shared, and where we curl up together for our favorite movies, wrapped in warmth and laughter.

Thank you for the small desk by the window in my bedroom, my little sanctuary for journaling and reflection, where morning sunlight and fresh air inspire my thoughts and dreams.

Thank you for my backyard patio, a retreat where I unwind under the stars, listening to the symphony of the night, and where weekend barbecues bring friends and family together in joyous celebration.

Thank you for my children's bedrooms, lovingly decorated to reflect their personalities, where they embark on nightly adventures in dreamland and wake up to a space that's uniquely theirs.

Thank you for the dining room table that has witnessed so many family dinners, where we share our day's highs and lows over plates of nourishing food, building a bond that strengthens with each shared meal.

Thank you for the cozy reading nook we created in the corner of the living room, where the kids lose themselves in books, surrounded by soft pillows and their favorite characters, fostering a lifelong love for reading.

Inhale deeply, embracing the warmth and comfort of home for a four-count: 1-2-3-4. Exhale slowly, releasing gratitude and kindness into the world. Repeat: inhale for 1-2-3-4, then gently exhale, feeling peace and calm. Continue this rhythm, feeling more relaxed with each breath.

Now we'll take a moment to give thanks for our natural world and environment.

Thank you for the majestic tree whose sturdy branches have inspired play for my children, with it's beautiful golden leaves in the fall.

Thank you for the small patch of wildflowers at the corner of the street, offering a splash of color and a reminder of nature's effortless beauty on my daily walks.

Thank you for the gentle stream that flows through the local park, where I find tranquility in its soothing sounds, a natural melody that eases my mind.

Thank you for the hummingbirds that visit my garden feeder, their delicate grace a delightful spectacle that reminds me of nature's intricate wonders.

Thank you for the starry nights that adorn the sky above my home, a vast canvas that inspires awe and puts life's worries into perspective.

Thank you for the first snowfall of the year, transforming the landscape into a winter wonderland, creating a sense of magic and wonder in the heart of my family.

Thank you for the sunsets that paint the horizon with vibrant hues, a daily masterpiece that signifies the end of one day and the promise of another.

Thank you for the refreshing rain, nurturing the earth around my home, bringing forth life and the fresh scent of renewal.

Breathe in deeply, filling your lungs with the fresh, clean air of nature, counting to four: 1-2-3-4. As you exhale, release your appreciation for the earth's beauty and bounty. Inhale again, 1-2-3-4, visualizing the vibrant life of forests, oceans, and skies. Exhale, expressing your gratitude and commitment to protect our planet. Continue this cycle, feeling a deeper connection to the environment with each breath.

Take a moment and let's send out our gratitude for some of our personal abilities and experiences.

Thank you for my ability to find humor in small things, turning everyday moments into pockets of joy and laughter.

Thank you for my capacity to empathize with others, allowing me to connect deeply and support those around me.

Thank you for my resilience in the face of adversity, transforming challenges into opportunities for growth and strength.

Thank you for the moments of clarity amidst chaos, guiding me to make decisions that align with my true self.

Thank you for the passion that drives my hobbies and interests, infusing my days with excitement and a sense of purpose.

Thank you for my creative sparks, whether in cooking, gardening, or crafting, which bring a unique flavor to my life and those around me.

Thank you for the quiet moments of introspection, where I can connect with my inner self and find peace and direction.

Thank you for the ability to learn from every person I meet, each one offering a different perspective and wisdom that enrich my understanding of the world.

Thank you for my sense of adventure, always nudging me towards new experiences and broadening my horizons.

Thank you for the moments of profound gratitude, where I truly feel the fullness of everything I have and am.

Thank you for the courage to step outside my comfort zone, leading to unexpected joys and learning.

Thank you for the gift of storytelling, allowing me to share experiences, wisdom, and laughter with those around me.

Thank you for my innate curiosity, which keeps the flame of learning and exploring forever alive in my heart.

Thank you for my ability to show kindness and compassion, creating ripples of positivity in the world.

Thank you for the quiet confidence that has grown over the years, guiding me with a gentle strength in my endeavors.

Thank you for my parent's love and nurturing, a constant source of comfort and strength in every step of my journey.

Thank you for the pure, unfiltered joy my children bring into my life, reminding me of the wonder and excitement of seeing the world through fresh eyes.

Thank you for the unique bond with each family member, and the love, learning, and shared memories that shape who I am.

Thank you for the person I am today, a culmination of experiences, lessons, and growth that have shaped my identity and values.

Thank you for the person I am becoming, continually evolving and embracing change, guided by aspirations and a vision for the future.

Thank you for the journey of self-discovery, where each step reveals new facets of my character and potential.

Thank you for the resilience and adaptability I have developed, crucial traits that empower me to navigate life's complexities with grace and strength.

Yes. Feels good. And breath in 1-2-3-4, and out. Breath in 1-2-3-4, and out. Inhale slowly, cherishing your unique abilities and experiences, counting steadily: 1-2-3-4. As you exhale, release any self-doubt, appreciating your journey and growth. Inhale again, 1-2-3-4, acknowledging the lessons learned and skills acquired. Exhale, feeling thankful for the challenges that have shaped you. Continue this rhythm, embracing gratitude for your personal journey with each breath.

Now we'll spend some time to give thanks for our interpersonal relationships and social aspects of our lives.

Thank you for the deep conversations with close friends that nourish my soul and broaden my perspectives.

Thank you for the unwavering support of my family, a foundation of love and understanding that grounds me.

Thank you for the laughter shared with colleagues, turning mundane moments into memories and strengthening our bonds.

Thank you for the wisdom imparted by mentors, guiding lights in my personal and professional growth.

Thank you for the kindness of strangers, small acts that restore faith in humanity and interconnectedness.

Thank you for the comfort of old friendships, enduring connections that stand the test of time and distance.

Thank you for the ability to forge new relationships, opening doors to diverse experiences and mutual enrichment.

Thank you for the moments of reconciliation, where forgiveness and understanding pave the way for renewed connections.

Thank you for the heartwarming family gatherings that bring us together, celebrating our unity and shared heritage.

Thank you for the empathetic ears of friends who listen without judgment, offering comfort in times of need.

Thank you for the joyous occasions shared with loved ones, milestones that weave the fabric of our collective lives.

Thank you for the spontaneous encounters that blossom into meaningful friendships, reminding us of life's delightful surprises.

Thank you for the community groups that foster a sense of belonging and purpose, uniting us in common causes and interests.

Thank you for the honest feedback from peers, a catalyst for self-improvement and personal growth.

Thank you for the heartfelt affection from pets, their unconditional love enriching our daily lives.

Thank you for the cultural traditions that connect us to our roots, offering a sense of identity and continuity.

Inhale deeply, drawing in the richness of your relationships and social connections, count slowly: 1-2-3-4. Exhale, releasing any feelings of loneliness or disconnect, and feel the warmth of companionship. Breathe in again, 1-2-3-4, cherishing memories and moments shared with others. Exhale, spreading feelings of love and gratitude outward. Continue this pattern, feeling your appreciation for social bonds deepen with each breath.

Now we'll give thanks for lifestyle and leisure.

Thank you for the peaceful walks in nature, where tranquility and the beauty of the outdoors rejuvenate my spirit.

Thank you for the books that transport me to other worlds, expanding my imagination and knowledge.

Thank you for the hobby that fills my time with joy and fulfillment, whether it's painting, gardening, or playing music.

Thank you for the vacations that provide a change of scenery and a break from routine, offering new experiences and relaxation.

Thank you for the exercise routines that keep my body healthy and my mind clear, be it yoga, jogging, or cycling.

Thank you for the quiet evenings spent at home, offering a haven for rest and personal reflection.

Thank you for the cultural events and performances that enrich my life with art, music, and creativity.

Thank you for the weekends, a pause from work, allowing time to indulge in leisure and connect with loved ones.

Thank you for the quiet moments with a cup of tea and a good book, a simple pleasure that offers escape and tranquility.

Thank you for the exhilarating hikes in the mountains, where the beauty of nature and the challenge of the climb invigorate my soul.

Thank you for the playful moments with my pet, whose antics and unconditional love bring daily joy and laughter into my life.

Thank you for the weekend gardening, where tending to plants and watching them grow brings a unique sense of achievement and connection to nature.

Thank you for the spontaneous road trips with friends, filled with music, conversation, and the freedom of the open road.

Thank you for the quiet early mornings spent in meditation or reflection, moments that ground me and set a peaceful tone for the day ahead.

Inhale slowly and deeply, absorbing the joys and comforts of your lifestyle and leisure, counting to four: 1-2-3-4. Hold this breath, savoring these moments of peace and enjoyment, for a six-count: 1-2-3-4-5-6. Gently exhale, releasing any stress or restlessness, feeling relaxation and contentment. Breathe in again, 1-2-3-4, immersing yourself in gratitude for life's pleasures. Hold, 1-2-3-4-5-6, then exhale slowly. With each cycle, deepen your appreciation for the simple joys in life.

And finally we'll conclude with our own avalanche of appreciation for our inner and emotional well-being.

Thank you for the moments of inner peace during meditation, where my mind is clear and my heart is calm, offering a sanctuary from life's hustle.

Thank you for the joy of laughter, a contagious spark that lightens my spirit and connects me with the happiness of the present moment.

Thank you for the tears that come with deep emotion, a cathartic release that cleanses and heals the soul.

Thank you for the ability to forgive, both myself and others, opening the path to healing and understanding.

Thank you for the personal growth from challenges faced, each one molding me into a stronger and wiser individual.

Thank you for the self-compassion I'm learning to practice, treating myself with kindness and understanding in times of struggle.

Thank you for the moments of deep gratitude that fill me with an overwhelming sense of abundance and fulfillment.

Thank you for the quiet confidence that has been growing within me, guiding my actions and decisions with a gentle assurance.

Thank you for the moments of spiritual alignment, where I feel deeply connected to a greater purpose and the universe itself, offering a profound sense of belonging and understanding.

Thank you for the practice of yoga and meditation, which open and balance my chakras, aligning my physical being with my spiritual essence.

Thank you for the experiences that have led to the awakening of my kundalini energy, revealing deeper layers of consciousness and spiritual enlightenment.

Thank you for the practice of tai chi and qigong, harmonizing my chi (qi) energy, and bringing a sense of balance and fluidity to my body and mind.

Thank you for the moments of deep intuition, where I feel guided by an inner wisdom that transcends logic, connecting me to a higher truth.

Thank you for the grounding practices that keep me centered and balanced, allowing me to navigate life's ups and downs with equanimity and grace.

Thank you for the insights gained through mindful practices, which bring clarity and peace to my mind, opening the path to self-discovery and inner harmony.

Thank you for the journey of spiritual growth, a path filled with learning, understanding, and the continuous evolution of my soul.

And now let's take a nice long cleansing breadth and give thanks for the easy, restful, restorative sleep we're about to allow ourselves.

Thank you for the quiet and serene environment that surrounds me, a haven for rest.

Thank you for the comfortable bed and pillows, cradling me into a state of relaxation.

Thank you for the day that has passed, with its lessons and experiences, now easing into night.

Thank you for the darkness that signals my body and mind to unwind and embrace tranquility.

Thank you for the peace within and around me, fostering deep and restful sleep.

Thank you for the opportunity to let go of stress and enter a realm of serene dreams.

Thank you for the promise of rejuvenation and healing that this night's sleep brings.

Thank you for the coming dawn, symbolizing a new beginning after a night of restful slumber.

Thank you for the gentle heaviness descending upon my eyelids, signaling the readiness for rest.

Thank you for each yawn that deepens my relaxation, drawing me closer to the world of dreams.

Thank you for the comforting weight settling in my body, a sign of the day's end and the night's embrace.

Thank you for the softness of the pillow and the warmth of the blanket, cocooning me in comfort.

Thank you for the quiet of the night, a peaceful backdrop to my journey into sleep.

Thank you for the sense of calm pervading my mind, clearing the way for serene slumber.

Thank you for the gradual release of all thoughts, allowing a tranquil and restorative sleep.

Thank you for the night's promise of rest, a rejuvenating pause in the rhythm of life.

Wonderful. And thank you for joining us in this gratitude sleep meditation.

As we resonate with gratitude we allow ourselves to drift off to sleep.

Like Ecclesiastes 3:1 says, "To everything there is a season, and a time to every purpose under the heaven." And this verse talks about there being a time to laugh, a time to dance, a time to keep silence, a time to love ..." And I would imagine, if I may, there is also "a time to sleep." And that time is now. Good night.

12

Gratitude Sleep Music

If you're listening to the audio version, you'll hear a segment of white noise with 528 Hz binaural beats for better sleep.

13

3 Short 10 Minute Sleep Meditations

This chapter gives you three quick and effective 10-minute meditations specifically for those who seek a swift transition into a restful slumber. Whether you're pressed for time, need a quick relaxation fix before bed, or simply prefer shorter meditation sessions, these practices are designed to cater to your needs.

The first of these short meditations is a Fast Relaxation Meditation for Slumber. This meditation is perfect for those who want to unwind quickly and prepare their mind and body for sleep. In just 10 minutes, you'll be guided through a series of relaxation techniques that will help you let go of the day's tensions and ease into a peaceful state.

The second short meditation is a Cognitive Behavioral Therapy for Insomnia (CBT-I) Guided Meditation for Restful Sleep. Drawing from Cognitive Behavioral Therapy for Insomnia (CBT-I) principles, this meditation is designed to address the cognitive and behavioral aspects of sleeplessness. It's a structured practice that will help you reframe negative sleep thoughts and relax your body, setting the stage for a good night's rest.

CBT-I is a structured and evidence-based approach to treating insomnia. It focuses on identifying and changing the thoughts and behaviors that contribute to sleep difficulties. Unlike medication, which can provide temporary relief, CBT-I aims to address the root causes of insomnia, providing long-term solutions.

CBT-I typically involves several components starting with Cognitive Restructuring. This involves identifying and challenging negative thoughts and beliefs about sleep, such as "I'll never be able to sleep well" or "I need 8 hours of sleep to function." By reframing these thoughts into more positive and realistic ones, individuals can reduce anxiety and improve their mindset towards sleep.

Behavioral Interventions is another important element of CBT-I. Behavioral Interventions include techniques such as stimulus control and sleep restriction. Stimulus control involves creating a strong association between the bed and sleep by limiting activities in bed to only sleep and sex. Sleep restriction involves limiting the amount of time spent in bed to match the actual time spent sleeping, which can increase sleep efficiency.

Relaxation Techniques such as progressive muscle relaxation, deep breathing, and guided imagery are often incorporated into CBT-I to help reduce physical tension and calm the mind. Many practitioners also include good Sleep Hygiene as part of their practice. This involves making lifestyle changes to promote better sleep, such as maintaining a regular sleep schedule, creating a comfortable sleep environment, and avoiding caffeine and electronics before bed.

CBT-I has been shown to be effective for many individuals with insomnia, often providing more lasting relief than medication. It can be particularly beneficial for those whose insomnia is driven by anxiety, stress, or negative thought patterns about sleep. By addressing both the cognitive and behavioral aspects of sleeplessness, CBT-I can help individuals develop healthier sleep habits and attitudes, leading to improved sleep quality and overall well-being.

The third short meditation is based on a powerful 2 Minute Military Method to Fall Asleep. Despite its name, this meditation extends the renowned 2-minute military technique into a 10-minute practice, allowing you to fully immerse in the process of relaxing your body and clearing your mind. It's a powerful method that has been used to help soldiers fall asleep quickly in challenging environments.

Each meditation is crafted to be accessible and straightforward, making it easy for you to incorporate them into your nightly routine. So, set aside just 10 minutes, find a comfortable spot, and let these meditations guide you into a restful and rejuvenating sleep.

The 2 Minute Military Method to Fall Asleep is a technique that was developed by the US military to help soldiers quickly fall asleep in challenging environments, such as on the battlefield or in other high-stress situations. The method was designed to ensure that soldiers could remain well-rested and alert, which is crucial for their performance and safety.

The method involves a series of relaxation steps that target different parts of the body, combined with controlled breathing and mental visualization. By systematically relaxing the muscles, starting from the arms and moving down to the legs, the body is prepared for sleep. The relaxation of the face, neck, and shoulders helps to release tension, which is often a barrier to falling asleep.

The mental aspect of the method is equally important. Focusing on slow, calming breaths helps to quiet the mind, while imagining a relaxing scene or repeating "Don't think, don't think, don't think" for 10 seconds helps to prevent intrusive thoughts that can disrupt the onset of sleep.

The history of this method is rooted in the military's recognition of the importance of sleep for the well-being and effectiveness of its personnel. Developed during World War II, it was included in a training program to help pilots relax and sleep under stressful conditions. The method proved to be effective, with reports suggesting that up to 96% of pilots were able to fall asleep within two minutes after six weeks of practice.

Today, the 2 Minute Military Method is not only used by soldiers but has also gained popularity among civilians looking for a quick and effective way to fall asleep. Its simplicity and effectiveness make it a valuable tool for anyone struggling with sleep issues.

Each of these short 10 minute meditations offers a unique approach to relaxation for sleep, allowing you to choose the method that best suits your needs. Now, sit back, relax, and let these meditations guide you into a peaceful and restorative slumber.

Fast Relaxation Meditation for Slumber (10 Minutes)

Welcome to this Fast Relaxation Meditation for Slumer, designed to quickly lead you into a deeper sleep. Let's start by getting comfortable in your bed. Find a position that feels natural for sleep, and gently close your eyes. Allow yourself to settle into the mattress, feeling supported and at ease.

Begin by taking a few deep breaths. Inhale deeply through your nose, feeling your chest and abdomen expand. Hold the breath for a moment, then exhale slowly through your mouth, releasing any tension you might be holding. Let each breath help you relax more deeply, inviting a sense of calm throughout your body.

Now, imagine a wave of relaxation starting at the top of your head. With each exhale, this wave gently flows down your body, bringing a soothing sensation to every area it touches. Feel it moving over your forehead, relaxing the muscles around your eyes, and softening any tension in your jaw.

Allow this wave of relaxation to continue down your neck and shoulders. With each breath, feel the tension melting away, as if you're releasing the weight of the day. The wave moves effortlessly, bringing comfort and ease to your chest, arms, and hands.

As we continue, feel the wave of relaxation flowing down to your abdomen and lower back. With each breath, your core relaxes, releasing any held tension, and allowing your body to sink deeper into the mattress. Embrace the sensation of warmth and comfort as it spreads through your body.

Now, let this wave of relaxation move further down to your hips and thighs. Feel the muscles in your legs loosening, becoming soft and heavy. With every exhale, imagine any remaining stress or discomfort flowing out through your toes, leaving your body completely relaxed and at peace.

As your body becomes more and more relaxed, allow your mind to follow. Visualize yourself gently drifting down into a deep, restful sleep. Imagine each breath taking you closer to the dreamy state of REM sleep, where your body can fully restore and rejuvenate.

Focus on the rhythm of your breathing, feeling it become more gentle and effortless. With each breath, you're moving closer to the healing, restorative phase of sleep. Allow yourself to let go, trusting that your body knows how to find its way to deep, restful slumber.

As you continue to relax deeply, imagine yourself gently transitioning into the stages of N3 non-rapid eye movement (NREM) sleep. This is a phase of progressively deeper sleep, where your body begins its important work of healing and restoration.

With each breath, feel yourself sinking deeper into this restorative state. Visualize your body repairing and regrowing tissues, building bone and muscle, and strengthening your immune system. Each cell in your body is rejuvenating, preparing you for the day ahead.

During this deep stage of NREM sleep, your breathing becomes even slower and more rhythmic. Your heart rate and blood pressure decrease, allowing your entire body to relax fully. Feel the sense of peace and safety as your body does its healing work.

Embrace the stillness and quiet of this deep sleep phase. Your mind is calm, and your body is completely at ease. With each moment, you're moving deeper into a state of restful, rejuvenating sleep, where your body can fully recharge.

As you journey deeper into the healing embrace of sleep, imagine your body's restorative processes working harmoniously. Every cell is bathed in a gentle glow of renewal, repairing any damage and fortifying your health.

Visualize your muscles relaxing completely, releasing any remaining tension. They are becoming stronger and more resilient as they rest. Your bones are absorbing essential nutrients, becoming denser and more robust.

Your immune system is working quietly but powerfully, warding off potential threats and keeping you protected. Feel a sense of gratitude for this intricate system that keeps you healthy and strong.

Now, let your mind drift into a state of complete relaxation. Allow any remaining thoughts to fade away, like wisps of cloud dissolving in a clear sky. Your mind is clear, calm, and ready for the deepest phase of sleep.

As we approach the end of this meditation, feel yourself fully embraced by the comforting arms of sleep. Every part of your body is relaxed, and your mind is at peace. You are in a safe and nurturing space, where you can let go and surrender to the restorative power of sleep.

With each gentle breath, allow yourself to drift further into the realm of dreams. Your journey through the night is one of healing and rejuvenation. Trust that your body knows exactly what it needs to do to restore balance and vitality.

Imagine yourself floating on a cloud of serenity, gently carried away into the depths of sleep. There is nothing more you need to do, nothing more you need to think about. Just let go and allow the natural rhythm of sleep to take over.

As this meditation comes to a close, carry this sense of relaxation and peace with you into your sleep. May your rest be deep and healing, and may you awaken feeling refreshed and renewed.

Goodnight, and sweet dreams.

CBT-I Guided Meditation for Restful Sleep (10 Minutes)

Welcome to this CBT-I Guided Meditation for Restful Sleep. Over the next 10 minutes, we'll focus on cognitive restructuring, a key component of Cognitive Behavioral Therapy for Insomnia. This practice will help you address and reframe negative thoughts about sleep, creating a more positive mindset for restful slumber.

To begin, find a comfortable position in your bed. Lie on your back or in any position that feels most comfortable for you. Gently close your eyes and take a few deep breaths. Inhale slowly through your nose, filling your lungs with air, and exhale gently through your mouth. With each breath, feel your body becoming more relaxed and at ease.

Now, let's bring attention to your thoughts about sleep. You may have thoughts like "I'll never be able to sleep well" or "I need a perfect night's sleep to function." Acknowledge these thoughts without judgment, and then gently let them go with your next exhale.

As you continue to relax and breathe deeply, let's focus on cultivating healthier sleep hygiene habits. Visualize yourself setting a consistent bedtime and wake-up time, creating a regular sleep schedule that supports your body's natural rhythm.

Imagine yourself preparing for bed each night by winding down with a relaxing routine. See yourself turning off electronic devices, dimming the lights, and maybe reading a book or taking a warm bath. Feel the sense of calm and readiness for sleep that these activities bring.

Now, picture your sleeping environment. Visualize your bedroom as a sanctuary for sleep, with comfortable bedding, a cool temperature, and a quiet, dark atmosphere. See yourself lying in bed, feeling safe and secure in this sleep-conducive environment.

Acknowledge the importance of avoiding caffeine and heavy meals close to bedtime. Imagine yourself choosing a light snack or a soothing herbal tea instead, making choices that support your body's readiness for sleep.

Next, we'll start the process of cognitive restructuring. Imagine these negative sleep thoughts are like leaves floating on a stream. Visualize yourself picking up each leaf, examining it, and then placing it back on the water to float away. As you do this, we'll begin to replace these thoughts with more positive, sleep-promoting affirmations.

As you continue to breathe deeply and comfortably, let's replace those negative sleep thoughts with positive affirmations. For each negative thought you identified, create a positive counter-statement. For example, if you thought "I'll never be able to sleep well," you can replace it with "I am learning to relax and improve my sleep."

Take a moment to think of a positive affirmation for each negative thought. As you do this, imagine writing these new, positive statements on the leaves floating in the stream. See them gliding away, carrying your new beliefs about sleep.

Now, repeat these positive affirmations to yourself, either silently or out loud. With each affirmation, visualize the words sinking into your mind, planting seeds of positive change. Feel the shift in your mindset as you focus on these encouraging and supportive thoughts.

Continue to breathe slowly and deeply, allowing these positive affirmations to resonate within you. With each breath, feel a sense of calm and confidence growing, as you embrace a more positive outlook on your sleep.

As you continue to breathe deeply and calmly, let's introduce some positive affirmations to replace those negative thoughts. When you notice a thought like "I'll never be able to sleep well," gently replace it with "Each night, I give my body the opportunity to rest and rejuvenate."

If you find yourself thinking, "I need a perfect night's sleep to function," replace it with "My body knows how to rest, and even a few hours of sleep can be refreshing." Feel the shift in your mindset as you embrace these more positive and forgiving thoughts.

With each affirmation, imagine yourself absorbing the positive energy of the words, letting them fill you with a sense of peace and confidence in your ability to sleep. Picture these affirmations as soothing light, gently enveloping your body and mind, creating a warm and comforting environment for sleep.

Now, let's focus on another common thought: "If I don't sleep well tonight, tomorrow will be ruined." Replace this with "Each day is a new opportunity, and I can handle whatever comes my way, regardless of how I slept." Feel the weight of pressure lifting off your shoulders as you embrace this more flexible and resilient perspective.

As we approach the end of this meditation, allow yourself to fully embrace the sense of relaxation and readiness for sleep that you've cultivated. Feel the comfort of your bed and the gentle rhythm of your breath, guiding you closer to sleep.

Let go of any remaining tension in your body, allowing yourself to sink deeper into the mattress. With each breath, feel a wave of relaxation sweeping over you, from the top of your head to the tips of your toes.

Now, gently release your focus on the meditation and allow your mind to drift. If thoughts arise, acknowledge them and then let them float away, returning to the sensation of your breath and the warmth of your bed.

Trust in the natural process of falling asleep. Your body knows how to rest and rejuvenate. Allow yourself to be carried into a peaceful and restorative sleep.

Goodnight and sweet dreams.

Revisit this meditation whenever they need assistance quieting any dialog concerning sleep in your head, or improving sleep hygiene habits.

2 Minute Military Method to Fall Asleep (10 Minutes)

Welcome to the 2 Minute Military Method to Fall Asleep, extended to a 10-minute meditation for a deeper relaxation experience. This method, originally developed for soldiers to quickly fall asleep in challenging environments, can help you find restful sleep in the comfort of your own home.

To begin, find a comfortable position lying on your back in your bed, chair, or meditation pillow. Allow your arms to rest gently by your sides, and make sure your legs are slightly apart. If you need to adjust your pillow or blankets, do so now to ensure you're as comfortable as possible.

Take a deep breath in through your nose, feeling your chest and belly rise. Hold it for a moment, and then slowly exhale through your mouth, letting all the tension leave your body. Repeat this deep breathing for a few more cycles, each time sinking deeper into relaxation.

Now, let's start the relaxation process. Focus on the top of your right arm. Gently tense your right biceps, feeling the muscles engage, and then slowly release, letting all the tension melt away. Move down to your right forearm, repeating the process: tense and then relax. Finally, focus on your right hand, tensing your fingers and then letting them go completely limp.

As you relax each part of your right arm, imagine the stress and tension draining away, leaving your muscles feeling heavy and relaxed. Take your time, and don't rush the process. The goal is to gradually release all the tension from your body.

Continue to breathe slowly and deeply as you relax each muscle group. With every exhale, feel yourself sinking deeper into the bed, becoming more and more relaxed.

Now, let's focus on your left arm. Begin with your left biceps, tensing the muscles gently, then slowly releasing them, allowing all tension to dissipate. Move down to your left forearm, repeating the process: tense and then relax. Lastly, turn your attention to your left hand, tensing your fingers before letting them relax completely.

Feel the relaxation spreading through your left arm, each muscle becoming heavier and more at ease. Allow this sense of calm to flow from your shoulders down to your fingertips.

Next, let's relax your face. Start with your forehead, imagining any lines of tension smoothing out as you relax the muscles. Move down to your eyes, allowing them to gently close if they haven't already. Relax your cheeks, your mouth, and finally, your jaw, letting go of any tightness or clenching.

As you continue to breathe deeply and evenly, imagine a wave of relaxation cascading down from the top of your head, through your face, and down your neck. Feel the muscles in your neck and shoulders releasing, becoming soft and relaxed. Let this wave of relaxation continue to spread, bringing a sense of peace and calm to your entire body.

Now, let's bring relaxation to your torso. Take a deep breath in, filling your chest and belly with air. As you exhale, feel any tension in your chest and abdomen melting away. Let this relaxation spread to your back, releasing any tightness in your upper, middle, and lower back.

With each breath, imagine your torso becoming lighter and more at ease. Feel the sense of calm deepening, as if you're floating on a gentle wave of tranquility.

Next, turn your attention to your hips and pelvis. Gently tense these muscles, then release, allowing them to sink into the bed. Feel the relaxation spreading through this area, releasing any stored tension or discomfort.

Now, focus on your legs. Start with your thighs, tensing them slightly, then relaxing them completely. Move down to your knees, calves, and finally your feet. Tense and relax each muscle group in turn, feeling the relaxation flow down your legs like a soothing stream.

As you relax your legs, imagine any remaining tension draining away through your toes, leaving your entire body feeling heavy, relaxed, and deeply at ease.

Now that your body is deeply relaxed, let's focus on calming your mind. Take a slow, deep breath in, filling your lungs with air. As you exhale, imagine any lingering thoughts or worries gently floating away, leaving your mind clear and serene.

Continue to take slow, calming breaths, feeling your body sink deeper into relaxation with each exhale. If any thoughts begin to intrude, gently acknowledge them and then let them go, returning your focus to your breath.

Now, imagine yourself sinking into the bed or chair, feeling completely supported and at ease. Visualize a warm, comforting light enveloping your body, further deepening your sense of relaxation and safety.

As you continue to breathe slowly and deeply, remind yourself that this time is for you to rest and rejuvenate. There's nothing else you need to do right now, no problems to solve or tasks to complete. Give yourself permission to let go and embrace the peace of the present moment.

As your body continues to relax, let's focus on clearing your mind. Take a slow, deep breath in, and as you exhale, imagine any remaining thoughts or worries gently floating away. With each breath, your mind becomes more peaceful and still.

If any thoughts do arise, acknowledge them without judgment and let them drift away like clouds in the sky. Return your focus to your breath, feeling the rise and fall of your chest and belly. Each breath takes you deeper into relaxation.

Now, visualize a place that brings you a sense of peace and calm. It could be a quiet beach, a serene forest, or any other place that feels safe and relaxing to you. Imagine yourself there, surrounded by tranquility and comfort.

With each breath, feel yourself becoming more and more immersed in this peaceful scene. Let the sense of calm and serenity fill your entire being.

As we come to the final moments of this meditation, allow yourself to sink even deeper into relaxation. Feel the weight of your body gently supported by your bed, completely at ease.

Take a few more slow, deep breaths, savoring the feeling of calm and relaxation that envelops you. With each exhale, let go of any remaining tension, sinking deeper into the comfort of your bed.

Now, gently release your focus on your breath and the visualization. Allow yourself to drift into the natural rhythm of your own breathing, letting it guide you into sleep.

There's nothing more you need to do or think about. Trust in the natural process of falling asleep. Let go and allow yourself to be carried into a restful and rejuvenating sleep.

Goodnight and sweet dreams.

14

Why Sleep Matters

Sleep is a cornerstone to life. Like eating or breathing, it's necessary. Unfortunately we can't just replace a battery, and then keep going - at least not yet.

Although there are a few animals that may not technically sleep, like upside-down jellyfish or bullfrogs. And while there are some that go long periods without sleep like whales and dolphins, others like giraffes and fruit flies naturally sleep only for extremely short periods. Humans, on the other hand, need a bare minimum of 4 hours of sleep by most estimates.

As of the writing of this book, the world record for going without sleep was 18 days, 21 hours, and 40 minutes. Robert McDonald achieved the Guinness World Record for the longest period of awareness in 1986.[7] Also of note was the record Randy Gardner set in 1963 for going 11 days and 25 minutes without sleep. Randy was 17-years-old at the time.[8]

---

[7] Coren, Stanley (1 March 2000). "Sleep Deprivation, Psychosis and Mental Efficiency". Psychiatric Times. 15 (3). Retrieved 2018-03-22.

[8] Keating, Sarah. "The boy who stayed awake for 11 days". www.bbc.com.

The amount of sleep a person needs can vary depending on numerous factors, including age, lifestyle, and individual differences. However, general guidelines have been established by organizations like the National Sleep Foundation.[9] Here's a breakdown based on age:

- Newborns and infants (0-11 months) need 12-17 hours of sleep each day.
- Toddlers and preschoolers (1-5 years) should get 10-14 hours of sleep.
- School-age children and teenagers (6-17 years) require 8-11 hours of sleep.
- Young adults and adults (18-64 years) need 7-9 hours of sleep, though some may need as little as 6 hours or as much as 10-11 hours.
- Older adults (65+ years) should get 7-8 hours of sleep.

It's important to note that while these are general guidelines, individual needs may differ. Some people feel refreshed and alert with just 6 hours of sleep, while others may need 10 hours to function optimally.

Nonetheless there seems to be no getting around the fact that humans need sleep to live. One study showed approximately 8% of mortality from all causes can be linked to inadequate or poor sleep quality.[10]

---

[9] How Much Sleep Do You Really Need?, October 1, 2020, https://www.thensf.org/how-many-hours-of-sleep-do-you-really-need/

[10] "Getting Good Sleep Could Add Years to Your Life," American College of Cardiology,

Several factors can influence sleep needs:

Lifestyle and Health: Stress, physical activity levels, dietary habits, and overall health can impact how much sleep one requires.

Sleep Quality: It's not just about quantity. Quality matters, too. Undisturbed, deep sleep is more restorative than fragmented sleep.

Genetics: Some individuals have genetic variants that seem to allow them to function well on fewer hours of sleep.

Consistently depriving oneself of the necessary amount of sleep can have serious health implications, including cognitive impairments, weakened immune function, increased risk for chronic conditions like obesity, diabetes, and heart disease, as well as mood disorders like depression and anxiety.

It's essential to find a balance that suits one's individual needs and to prioritize sleep as a vital component of overall health and well-being.

Feb 23, 2023, https://www.acc.org/About-ACC/Press-Releases/2023/02/22/21/35/Getting-Good-Sleep-Could-Add-Years-to-Your-Life

15

Relaxation Exercises

Relaxation exercises are powerful tools that can help calm your mind and prepare your body for a restful night's sleep. These practices can be particularly beneficial if you find yourself struggling to unwind or if your thoughts tend to race as bedtime approaches. By incorporating techniques such as mindful breathing, counting breaths, and the 4-7-8 breathing method, you can create a sense of inner peace and tranquility. Progressive muscle relaxation and visualization of sleepiness further enhance this relaxation, allowing you to let go of physical tension and mental stress. Mantra repetition and autogenic training offer additional ways to focus your mind and induce a state of calm. Whether you're dealing with occasional sleeplessness or more persistent insomnia, these relaxation exercises can be a valuable part of your bedtime routine, guiding you gently towards a deep and rejuvenating sleep.

Following some of these relaxation techniques, you can explore various journaling practices and other strategies to further support your journey to a peaceful night's rest. These include gratitude journaling, reflective journaling, and pre-sleep brain dumps, which can help you process your day and clear your mind. Dream journaling, mood tracking, and setting intentions for the next day can also contribute to a more positive and relaxed mindset. Positive affirmations and sleep analysis provide additional tools to foster a conducive sleep environment. Lastly, letter writing can be a therapeutic way to release any lingering emotions or concerns, ensuring that you can rest with a lighter heart.

Mindful Breathing

Mindful breathing is a simple yet effective technique that can significantly improve the quality of your sleep. By focusing on the breath and practicing slow, deep breathing, you can calm the mind and relax the body, creating the ideal conditions for a restful night's sleep.

To practice mindful breathing for sleep, start by finding a comfortable position in bed. Close your eyes and take a moment to notice any areas of tension in your body. Gently shift your attention to your breath. Observe the natural rhythm of your inhalation and exhalation without trying to change it. Simply be aware of the sensation of air entering and leaving your body.

As you become more attuned to your breathing, begin to deepen your breaths. Inhale slowly through your nose, allowing your chest and abdomen to expand. Then, exhale gently through your mouth, making each exhale a little longer than the inhale. This pattern of breathing helps activate the body's relaxation response, signaling to your nervous system that it's time to unwind.

Continue to focus on your breath, letting go of any distracting thoughts or worries. If your mind starts to wander, gently guide it back to the sensation of breathing. With each breath, imagine yourself sinking deeper into relaxation, releasing any remaining tension or stress.

Mindful breathing can be a powerful tool to quiet the mind and prepare the body for sleep. By practicing this technique regularly, you can enhance your ability to fall asleep more easily and enjoy a deeper, more restorative sleep.

Counting Breaths: Gently count your breaths. Count "one" as you inhale, "two" as you exhale, up to ten, and then start again at one. This helps keep your mind focused and prevents it from wandering.

4-7-8 Breathing Technique

The 4-7-8 Breathing Technique is a simple yet powerful breathing exercise that can promote relaxation and improve sleep quality. Developed by Dr. Andrew Weil, a renowned integrative medicine physician, this technique is based on pranayama, an ancient yogic practice that helps regulate the breath.[11] The 4-7-8 method is particularly effective for reducing anxiety and calming the nervous system, making it an excellent practice for those struggling to fall asleep.

To practice the 4-7-8 Breathing Technique for sleep, start by finding a comfortable position in bed. You can lie on your back with your hands resting gently on your abdomen or by your sides. Close your eyes and take a few natural breaths to settle into the moment.

Begin the exercise by exhaling completely through your mouth, making a whooshing sound. Then, close your mouth and inhale

[11] Andrew Weil, M.D., "Breathing: The Master Key to Self-Healing," (Boulder, CO: Sounds True, 1999).

quietly through your nose to a mental count of four. Hold your breath for a count of seven. Finally, exhale completely through your mouth, making the whooshing sound again, to a count of eight.

Repeat this breathing pattern for four full cycles. Inhale for four counts, hold for seven counts, and exhale for eight counts. With each cycle, allow yourself to become more relaxed and at ease. The specific counts in this technique help to slow down your breathing and heart rate, which in turn signals to your body that it's time to relax and prepare for sleep.

The 4-7-8 Breathing Technique can be a powerful tool in your sleep hygiene arsenal. By practicing this exercise regularly, you can train your body to release tension and stress more effectively, paving the way for a peaceful and restful night's sleep.

Progressive Muscle Relaxation

Progressive Muscle Relaxation (PMR) was developed by Dr. Edmund Jacobson in the early 20th century. Dr. Jacobson, an American physician and physiologist, introduced this technique in his book "Progressive Relaxation" published in 1929.[12] He believed that physical relaxation could lead to mental relaxation, and his research focused on the relationship between muscle tension and stress.

The premise of PMR is based on the observation that there is a close connection between physical tension and psychological stress. When the body is tense, it can signal the mind to be in a state of alertness or anxiety, making it difficult to relax or fall asleep.

---

[12] Edmund Jacobson, Progressive Relaxation (Chicago: University of Chicago Press, 1929).

Conversely, when the muscles are relaxed, it can promote a sense of mental calmness and reduce stress levels.

PMR is effective for sleep because it directly addresses one of the common barriers to falling asleep: physical tension. By systematically tensing and then relaxing each muscle group, the body is encouraged to enter a state of deep relaxation. This process not only helps to release built-up tension but also shifts the focus away from racing thoughts or worries that can interfere with sleep.

Additionally, the practice of PMR can activate the parasympathetic nervous system, which is responsible for the body's rest-and-digest functions. This activation can lower heart rate, reduce blood pressure, and promote a state of calmness, all of which are conducive to falling asleep and achieving restorative sleep.

To practice Progressive Muscle Relaxation exercises for sleep, start by lying down in a comfortable position in bed. Close your eyes and take a few deep breaths to center yourself. Begin with your toes and feet. Tense the muscles in this area as tightly as you can for a few seconds, then release the tension and notice the feeling of relaxation that follows. Pay attention to the contrast between the tension and the relaxation, as this awareness can enhance the relaxation experience.

Continue this process with each muscle group in your body, moving upward. Tense your calf muscles, hold for a few seconds, and then relax. Move on to your thighs, buttocks, abdomen, and so on, all the way up to your facial muscles. As you tense and relax each muscle group, focus on the sensation of release and the deepening relaxation that accompanies it.

When you reach your head, take a moment to relax your facial muscles, including your forehead, eyes, and jaw. Finally, take a few deep breaths, allowing your entire body to relax even further.

Progressive Muscle Relaxation can be a powerful tool for preparing your body and mind for sleep. By systematically releasing tension from each muscle group, you can create a state of deep relaxation that is conducive to falling asleep and staying asleep. Regular practice of PMR can improve your overall sleep quality and help you wake up feeling more refreshed and rejuvenated.

The history and principles of PMR highlight its effectiveness as a relaxation technique that can improve sleep quality by reducing physical tension and promoting mental relaxation.

Visualization of Sleepiness

The technique of Visualization of Sleepiness is rooted in the broader practice of guided imagery and visualization, which have been used for centuries in various cultures for relaxation and healing purposes. The specific application of visualizing sleepiness as a way to induce sleep is a more modern adaptation, influenced by the principles of relaxation therapy and cognitive-behavioral therapy.

The effectiveness of Visualization of Sleepiness lies in its ability to engage the mind in a focused and calming activity, shifting attention away from the stresses or worries that can interfere with sleep. By imagining sleep as a warm, comforting presence, the body responds by relaxing, which in turn, can make it easier to fall asleep.

This technique also taps into the mind-body connection, where mental imagery can have a direct impact on physical sensations. Visualizing a warm wave or substance moving through the body can induce a feeling of warmth and relaxation, which are physical states conducive to sleep.

Furthermore, Visualization of Sleepiness can help activate the parasympathetic nervous system, which is responsible for the body's rest-and-digest functions.[13] This activation promotes a state of calmness and relaxation, further facilitating the onset of sleep.

Visualization of Sleepiness is a powerful relaxation technique that can help ease the transition into sleep. By using the power of imagination, this practice encourages the body and mind to enter a state of deep relaxation and drowsiness, paving the way for a restful night's sleep.

To practice this technique, start by lying comfortably in bed, with your eyes closed. Take a few deep breaths to center yourself and release any initial tension. Begin to visualize sleep as a warm, gentle wave or a comforting, warm substance. Imagine it starting at your feet, slowly enveloping them with a sense of warmth and relaxation.

As this warm sensation rises, allow it to move up through your legs, relaxing your calves, knees, and thighs. Feel the muscles in your legs becoming heavier and more relaxed with each passing moment. Let this feeling of warmth and relaxation continue to spread upwards, reaching your hips, abdomen, and lower back. With each breath, imagine the wave of sleepiness rising higher, bringing a deeper sense of relaxation to every part of your body.

Visualize this comforting warmth moving up through your chest and shoulders, releasing any tension you may be holding in these

[13] Herbert Benson, The Relaxation Response (New York: HarperTorch, 1975).

areas. Feel your arms and hands becoming heavy and relaxed as the warmth envelops them. Allow the sensation to continue rising, reaching your neck and head. Imagine your facial muscles softening, your jaw releasing, and your mind becoming calm and peaceful.

As the warm wave of sleepiness reaches the top of your head, imagine your entire body being completely enveloped in this comforting warmth. Your body feels heavy, relaxed, and ready for sleep. Embrace this feeling of drowsiness and allow yourself to drift off into a deep, restful sleep.

Visualization of Sleepiness is an effective way to calm the mind and relax the body, making it an ideal practice for those who struggle to fall asleep. By focusing on the sensation of warmth and relaxation spreading through the body, you can gently guide yourself into a state of sleepiness and prepare for a night of rejuvenating rest.

Mantra Repetition

Mantras have a rich ancient history that dates back thousands of years, deeply rooted in various spiritual and religious traditions, including Hinduism and Buddhism. The word "mantra" originates from Sanskrit, with "man" meaning mind and "tra" meaning instrument or tool. Thus, a mantra is an instrument of the mind, a powerful sound or vibration that you can use to enter a deep state of meditation.

In Hinduism, mantras are considered sacred sounds or phrases that are believed to have spiritual and psychological power. They are often used in rituals, meditation, and prayer to invoke divine energy and connect with higher states of consciousness. In Buddhism, mantras are used as a form of meditation to cultivate qualities such as compassion, wisdom, and focus. The repetition of mantras is believed to help purify the mind, reduce negative emotions, and promote inner peace.

Mantras are powerful for sleep because they provide a simple yet effective way to focus the mind and induce a state of relaxation. When you repeat a calming word or phrase silently, it helps to quiet the chatter of the mind and create a sense of tranquility. This mental focus can shift your attention away from stress, worries, or racing thoughts that often interfere with sleep.

The rhythmic repetition of a mantra can also have a soothing effect on the nervous system, helping to activate the parasympathetic nervous system, which is responsible for the body's rest-and-digest functions. This relaxation response can lower heart rate, reduce blood pressure, and prepare the body for restful sleep.

Overall, the ancient practice of mantra repetition complements the principles of mindfulness and meditation found in Buddhism and other spiritual traditions. By focusing the mind on a calming word or phrase, you can create the ideal conditions for a peaceful and restorative night's sleep.

Mantra Repetition is a simple yet powerful meditation technique that involves silently repeating a calming word or phrase to focus the mind and induce a state of relaxation. This practice is rooted in various spiritual and religious traditions, where mantras are often used as a tool for meditation and mindfulness.

To practice Mantra Repetition for sleep, choose a word or phrase that evokes a sense of calm and tranquility. It could be a word like "peace," "relax," "let go," or any other soothing word that resonates with you. As you lie in bed, close your eyes and take a few deep breaths to settle into a relaxed state.

Begin to silently repeat your chosen mantra in your mind. With each repetition, allow yourself to sink deeper into relaxation. Focus solely on the sound and rhythm of the mantra, letting it anchor your mind and prevent it from wandering. If you find your thoughts drifting, gently guide your attention back to the mantra.

The repetition of a calming mantra can help quiet the internal chatter that often keeps us awake at night. By concentrating on a single word or phrase, you create a mental space that is conducive to relaxation and sleep. The rhythmic nature of the repetition can also have a soothing effect, similar to a lullaby, which can further promote a sense of drowsiness.

Mantra Repetition is an effective tool for those who struggle with racing thoughts or anxiety at bedtime. By providing a simple focal point for the mind, it can help ease the transition into sleep, leading to a more restful and rejuvenating night.

Autogenic Training

Autogenic Training is a self-relaxation technique developed in the early 20th century by German psychiatrist Johannes Heinrich Schultz.[14] It involves a series of exercises designed to induce a state of relaxation and reduce stress by focusing on physical sensations in the body. The technique is often used to improve sleep quality, as it promotes a state of calm and relaxation that is conducive to falling asleep.

---

[14] Johannes Heinrich Schultz, Das Autogene Training: Konzentrative Selbstentspannung (Stuttgart: Georg Thieme Verlag, 1932).

To practice Autogenic Training for sleep, you begin by finding a comfortable position in bed, lying on your back with your arms and legs slightly apart. Close your eyes and take a few deep breaths to center yourself. Then, start repeating calming phrases or suggestions in your mind, focusing on different parts of your body. For example, you might start by saying to yourself, "My arms and legs are heavy and warm." As you repeat this phrase, imagine your limbs becoming heavier and warmer, sinking into the bed.

Next, you might focus on your heartbeat, repeating a phrase like, "My heartbeat is calm and regular." Visualize your heart beating steadily, promoting a sense of inner peace. Continue with phrases that focus on your breathing, such as, "My breath is slow and even." Imagine your breath flowing gently in and out, further deepening your state of relaxation.

Autogenic Training works by tapping into the body's natural relaxation response, similar to self-hypnosis. By concentrating on physical sensations and repeating calming phrases, you can shift your attention away from anxious thoughts or worries that might keep you awake. This mental focus helps to quiet the mind and relax the body, making it easier to drift off into sleep.

The beauty of Autogenic Training is that it can be personalized to suit your individual needs. You can create your own phrases that resonate with you, focusing on areas of your body where you tend to hold tension. With regular practice, this technique can become a valuable part of your bedtime routine, helping you to achieve a deeper, more restful sleep.

Yoga Nidra

Yoga Nidra, often referred to as "yogic sleep," is a powerful meditation technique that originates from the ancient teachings of yoga. Unlike traditional yoga that focuses on physical postures, Yoga Nidra is a form of guided relaxation that aims to bring the practitioner into a deeply restful state, hovering between wakefulness and sleep. This practice is known for its profound restorative effects and has gained popularity as a method to manage insomnia and improve overall sleep quality.

This specialized type of Yoga has its roots in the ancient mystical traditions of India. It is a practice deeply embedded in the teachings of Tantra and Vedanta, which are branches of Indian philosophy that explore the nature of consciousness and the universe. The origins of Yoga Nidra can be traced back to the Upanishads, which are a collection of ancient sacred texts that form the basis of Hindu philosophy.

The Upanishads contain references to the states of consciousness and the practice of deep, dreamless sleep as a means of accessing higher states of awareness. Yoga Nidra is considered a form of Pratyahara, or withdrawal of the senses, which is one of the eight limbs of classical yoga outlined by the sage Patanjali in his Yoga Sutras.[15] In this practice, the individual withdraws from external stimuli and turns inward, exploring the depths of their own consciousness.

The Tantric tradition, which emerged around the middle of the first millennium CE, further developed the practice of Yoga Nidra.

---

[15] Patanjali, Yoga Sutras of Patanjali, translated by Swami Satchidananda (Buckingham, VA: Integral Yoga Publications, 2012), sutra 2.54-2.55.

Tantric texts describe techniques for entering into a state of deep meditation, where the practitioner remains aware while the body and mind are at rest. This state is seen as a gateway to experiencing the union of individual consciousness with universal consciousness, leading to spiritual awakening.

In modern times, the practice of Yoga Nidra has been popularized by teachers like Swami Satyananda Saraswati, founder of the Bihar School of Yoga. He systematized the practice in the mid-20th century, making it accessible to a wider audience. His approach to Yoga Nidra combines traditional yogic teachings with contemporary psychology, emphasizing its therapeutic benefits for physical and mental well-being.

The mystical origins of Yoga Nidra highlight its profound nature as a practice that goes beyond mere relaxation. It is a journey into the deepest layers of the self, offering a path to inner peace, self-discovery, and ultimately, a connection to the divine.

During a Yoga Nidra session, the practitioner lies comfortably on their back, typically supported by blankets or cushions to ensure complete relaxation. A guide or instructor then leads them through a series of relaxation techniques, starting with setting an intention or Sankalpa for the practice. This intention serves as a focal point and helps to deepen the meditative state.

The guide then directs the practitioner's attention to various parts of the body, often following a systematic rotation of consciousness. This body scan helps to release physical tension and promote a sense of bodily awareness. The practitioner is encouraged to remain in a state of passive observation, simply noticing sensations without trying to change them.

In addition to the body scan, Yoga Nidra may include visualization exercises, breath awareness, and techniques to cultivate a sense of detachment from thoughts and emotions. The goal is to reach a state of inner stillness and profound relaxation, where the mind becomes quiet and the body can deeply rest.

For example a beneficial pose for Yoga Nidra is Savasana, also known as Corpse Pose, which is a restorative yoga posture frequently used for relaxation and meditation. When practicing Savasana with palms facing up, the position is as follows. Begin by lying flat on your back on a yoga mat or a comfortable surface. Ensure that your spine is straight and your legs are extended. Allow your feet to fall naturally to the sides, about hip-width apart.

Then place your arms by your sides, keeping a slight distance between your arms and your torso. This allows your shoulders to relax and open. Turn your palms to face upward, towards the ceiling. This position of the palms is symbolic of openness and receptivity, allowing you to fully relax and receive the benefits of the pose. Make sure your head is in a neutral position, with your chin slightly tucked in. This ensures that your neck is in line with the rest of your spine. Use a small pillow or folded blanket under your head if you need support to maintain this alignment.

Close your eyes and take a few deep breaths to settle into the pose. With each exhale, allow your body to relax further into the ground. Let go of any tension in your muscles and focus on the sensation of your breath. Remain in Savasana for several minutes, allowing your body and mind to fully relax and rejuvenate. When you're ready to come out of the pose, gently wiggle your fingers and toes, and slowly roll to one side before pressing yourself up to a seated position.

Yoga Nidra is particularly effective for managing insomnia because it addresses both the physical and mental aspects of sleeplessness. By relaxing the body and calming the mind, it creates the ideal conditions for falling asleep. The deep relaxation experienced during Yoga Nidra can also improve sleep quality and increase the feeling of being well-rested upon waking.

Regular practice of Yoga Nidra can have a cumulative effect, helping to reduce stress levels, balance the nervous system, and promote a more peaceful state of being, all of which contribute to better sleep over time.

Gratitude Journaling

Gratitude journaling is a simple yet powerful practice that can have a profound impact on your overall well-being, especially when it comes to improving the quality of your sleep. By taking a few moments before bed to write down three to five things you are grateful for, you can shift your mindset from one of stress and worry to one of positivity and appreciation.

This shift in perspective is crucial for relaxation, as it helps to quiet the mind and ease any tension that might be lingering from the day. Focusing on gratitude brings your attention to the positive aspects of your life, which can naturally lead to a sense of contentment and peace. This emotional state is conducive to falling asleep more easily and enjoying a deeper, more restorative sleep.

Moreover, gratitude journaling can help break the cycle of negative thinking that often contributes to insomnia. By actively acknowledging the good in your life, you're training your brain to notice and appreciate the positive, rather than dwelling on the negative. This can reduce the stress and anxiety that often keep people awake at night.

In addition to its benefits for sleep, gratitude journaling has been linked to a range of other health benefits, including improved mood, increased resilience, and even better physical health. By incorporating this practice into your nightly routine, you're not only setting the stage for a good night's sleep but also contributing to your overall happiness and well-being.

Overall, gratitude journaling is a simple, yet effective tool for promoting relaxation and improving sleep quality. By ending your day with a focus on the positive, you can create a mindset that supports restful sleep and a more joyful life.

An example Gratitude Journal Entry might include the following.

***

Date: February 20, 2024

- *Family Support: Today, I am deeply grateful for the unwavering support of my family. Their love and encouragement give me strength and make me feel valued and understood.*
- *Health: I am thankful for my good health, which allows me to enjoy life's activities and pursue my goals with energy and vitality.*
- *Nature's Beauty: I am grateful for the beautiful sunset I witnessed this evening. The vibrant colors and peaceful atmosphere filled me with a sense of awe and tranquility.*

- *Friendship: I appreciate the laughter and meaningful conversation I shared with my friend today. It's a reminder of the joy and comfort that genuine connections bring to my life.*
- *Opportunities for Growth: I am thankful for the challenges I faced today, as they provided me with valuable learning experiences and opportunities for personal growth.*

***

Here are a few gratitude journal exercises specifically designed to promote relaxation and improve sleep:

End-of-Day Reflections: Before going to bed, take a few minutes to reflect on your day. Write down three to five things that you are grateful for from the day. These can be small moments, like enjoying a delicious cup of coffee, or bigger events, like receiving good news or spending time with loved ones.

Gratitude for Challenges: Write about a challenge you faced during the day and how it helped you grow or learn something new. Expressing gratitude for difficult experiences can help you reframe them positively and reduce stress.

Body Gratitude: Focus on your body and write down things you are grateful for about it. This could be its ability to heal, the strength it gives you to accomplish tasks, or the simple fact that it allows you to experience the world around you.

Gratitude for Sleep: Write about the aspects of sleep you are grateful for. This could be the comfort of your bed, the quiet of the night, or the opportunity to rest and recharge.

Future Gratitude: Write down things you are looking forward to in the future. Anticipating positive experiences can help create a sense of excitement and optimism, which can be calming and conducive to sleep.

Gratitude for Others: Reflect on the people in your life who have supported or positively impacted you. Write a note of thanks to someone who made your day better, even in a small way.

Sensory Gratitude: Pay attention to your senses and write down things you are grateful for that you can see, hear, touch, taste, and smell. This can help ground you in the present moment and foster a sense of appreciation for your surroundings.

By incorporating these gratitude journal exercises into your bedtime routine, you can cultivate a more positive mindset, reduce stress, and create a peaceful state of mind that is conducive to restful sleep.

Reflective Journaling

Reflective journaling is a therapeutic practice that involves writing down your thoughts, feelings, and experiences from the day. This form of journaling can be particularly beneficial before bed, as it allows you to process the events of the day, release any pent-up emotions, and clear your mind for a restful night's sleep.

When you engage in reflective journaling, you create a space to explore your inner world and gain insights into your emotions and reactions. By noting significant events, you can acknowledge and celebrate your achievements, no matter how small they may seem. This recognition can foster a sense of accomplishment and positivity.

Writing about your feelings is a key aspect of reflective journaling. It provides an outlet for expressing emotions that you may have suppressed during the day. Whether you're feeling joy, gratitude, sadness, or frustration, putting these emotions into words can help you understand and process them. This emotional release can reduce stress and anxiety, making it easier to relax and prepare for sleep.

Reflective journaling also allows you to explore your thoughts and beliefs. You can examine your thought patterns, challenge negative thinking, and reinforce positive self-talk. This mental clarity can help you let go of worries or concerns that might otherwise keep you awake at night.

To make the most of reflective journaling for sleep, try to write in a calm and comfortable setting. Use this time to wind down and transition from the busyness of the day to a more peaceful state of mind. You don't need to write for long—a few minutes may be enough to capture the essence of your day and release any lingering tension.

Here's an example of a reflective journal entry that can help with sleep:

***

Date: March 3, 2024

Today's Highlights:

- *Had a productive meeting at work where my project proposal was well-received.*
- *Enjoyed a lovely lunch with a colleague, which brightened my day.*
- *Completed a challenging workout in the evening, which felt invigorating.*

Feelings and Emotions:

- *I felt proud and appreciated after the positive feedback on my project proposal.*
- *Gratitude for the friendship and support of my colleague.*
- *A sense of accomplishment after pushing through my workout, even though I was initially reluctant.*

Challenges:

- *Felt a bit overwhelmed in the morning with the workload.*
- *Experienced some frustration with a technical issue that delayed my work.*

Reflections:

- *Recognizing the importance of taking breaks and not overloading myself. It's okay to ask for help when needed.*
- *The lunch with my colleague reminded me of the value of connecting with others and how it can uplift my mood.*
- *Proud of myself for not skipping the workout, as it ultimately boosted my energy and mood.*

Thoughts for Tomorrow:

- *Plan to start the day with a short meditation to set a positive tone.*
- *Need to follow up on the technical issue and seek assistance if it persists.*
- *Looking forward to a quiet evening at home to unwind and relax.*

Gratitude:

- *Thankful for the supportive work environment and the opportunities to grow.*
- *Grateful for my health and the ability to stay active.*
- *Appreciative of the small joys in life, like a good meal and laughter with a friend.*

***

Overall, reflective journaling is a powerful tool for self-discovery and emotional well-being. By incorporating this practice into your bedtime routine, you can create a sense of closure for the day, foster a positive mindset, and set the stage for a restful and rejuvenating night's sleep.

Pre-Sleep Brain Dump

The Pre-Sleep Brain Dump is a simple yet effective technique to help clear your mind before bed, promoting a more relaxed state conducive to sleep. This practice involves writing down any worries, to-do lists, or random thoughts that are occupying your mind, thereby transferring them from your mental space onto paper.

The act of writing down your thoughts can be therapeutic, as it provides a physical outlet for the mental clutter that often accumulates throughout the day. By externalizing your worries and tasks, you create a sense of order and control, which can reduce feelings of overwhelm and anxiety. This process can also help you identify specific concerns that may need attention, allowing you to address them more effectively during waking hours.

Creating a to-do list for the next day as part of your brain dump can also be beneficial. It allows you to organize your thoughts and priorities, ensuring that you have a clear plan of action when you wake up. This can reduce the mental load of trying to remember everything you need to do, allowing your mind to relax and prepare for sleep.

In addition to worries and tasks, you can also use the brain dump to jot down any creative ideas or insights that come to you before bed. This ensures that you won't forget them overnight and can explore them further when you're well-rested.

To practice a Pre-Sleep Brain Dump, keep a notebook and pen by your bedside. Spend a few minutes before turning off the lights to write down anything that's on your mind. Don't worry about organizing your thoughts or writing in complete sentences—the goal is simply to transfer your thoughts onto paper. Once you've emptied your mind, close the notebook and set it aside, giving yourself permission to let go of those thoughts until the morning.

By incorporating a Pre-Sleep Brain Dump into your nightly routine, you can create a mental space that's more conducive to relaxation and restful sleep. This practice can be a valuable tool in managing stress and improving overall sleep quality.

Here's a pre-sleep brain dump journal entry for example.

***

Date: July 12, 2023

Tired eyes blink against the soft glow of the lamp, mind racing like a jazz riff, thoughts tumbling and jiving, a chaotic symphony of the day's echoes. Need to remember to call Mom tomorrow, her voice a comforting melody in the cacophony of life. The project at work, looming like a mountain, deadlines dancing like shadows, gotta break it down, piece by piece, can't let it swallow me whole.

Grocery list scribbles itself in the corner of my mind, milk, eggs, bread, the essentials of survival in this urban jungle. The leaky faucet, a persistent drip-drip-drip, a reminder of tasks undone, a nagging itch in the back of my brain. Oh, and that book I've been meaning to read, its pages unturned, a universe undiscovered, must make time for that, escape into someone else's story for a while.

The weight of the world, heavy on my shoulders, news headlines screaming from the abyss, need to stay informed but not drown in the darkness. A flicker of inspiration, a poem perhaps, words swirling, a dance of light and shadow, must jot that down before it evaporates into the ether.

And then, there's tomorrow, a blank canvas, a fresh start, endless possibilities, but first, must navigate the landscape of dreams, find solace in the arms of Morpheus. Tonight, let the worries fade, the mind quiet, the body rest, for tomorrow is another journey, another chance to ride the wild rhythm of life.

***

Releasing such thoughts onto paper through a free-flowing stream of consciousness can be a liberating experience. It's like opening the floodgates of the mind, allowing the torrent of worries, ideas, and reflections to flow out, leaving behind a sense of calm and clarity.

This process of unburdening the mind can create a peaceful space for sleep to gently envelop you, guiding you into a restful slumber where the chaos of the day fades into the tranquility of the night. By embracing this cathartic release, you can drift off with a lighter heart and a clearer mind, ready to embrace the dreams that await in the quietude of sleep.

Dream Journaling

Dream journaling has a fascinating history, intertwined with the exploration of the subconscious mind and the interpretation of dreams. Sigmund Freud and Carl Jung are two of the most influential figures in the field of psychology who have contributed significantly to our understanding of dreams and their meanings.

Sigmund Freud, often referred to as the father of psychoanalysis, viewed dreams as a window into the unconscious mind. In his seminal work, "The Interpretation of Dreams," Freud proposed that dreams are a form of wish fulfillment, revealing our deepest desires and unresolved conflicts.[16] He believed that by analyzing the symbols and imagery in dreams, individuals could uncover hidden aspects of their psyche and address underlying issues.

Carl Jung, a contemporary and one-time collaborator of Freud, had a different perspective on dreams. Jung saw dreams as a means of communication between the conscious and unconscious mind, serving to guide and inform the individual. He introduced the concept of archetypes, universal symbols and themes that appear in dreams and are shared across cultures.[17] Jung believed that by understanding these archetypes, individuals could gain insight into their personal growth and development.

Ann Faraday, a psychologist and dream researcher, further popularized the practice of dream journaling in her book "The Dream Game." Faraday advocated for the use of a dream diary as a tool for

---

[16] Sigmund Freud, The Interpretation of Dreams, trans. James Strachey (New York: Basic Books, 2010).

[17] Carl G. Jung, Archetypes and the Collective Unconscious, in The Collected Works of C.G. Jung, vol. 9, part 1, ed. Herbert Read, Michael Fordham, and Gerhard Adler, trans. R.F.C. Hull (Princeton, NJ: Princeton University Press, 1981).

self-discovery and personal transformation.[18] She encouraged individuals to record their dreams in detail and explore their meanings through techniques such as free association and amplification.

The strange origins and imagery in dreams have long been a source of fascination and intrigue. Dream journaling provides a way to capture and reflect on these mysterious experiences, allowing individuals to delve into the depths of their subconscious and uncover the messages and insights that their dreams may hold. By exploring the symbolism and themes in their dreams, people can gain a better understanding of themselves and their inner world.

Dream journaling is a practice that involves keeping a journal near your bed to record your dreams as soon as you wake up. This habit can provide valuable insights into your subconscious mind, helping you to understand the hidden messages and themes in your dreams. By exploring the content of your dreams, you can gain a deeper understanding of your emotions, fears, desires, and unresolved issues.

Recording your dreams can also help reduce nighttime anxiety. When you write down your dreams, you externalize them, which can make them feel less overwhelming and easier to manage. This process can help you identify patterns or recurring themes in your dreams that may be linked to sources of stress or anxiety in your waking life. By addressing these underlying issues, you can reduce the frequency of anxiety-inducing dreams and improve your overall sleep quality.

To start dream journaling, keep a notebook and pen within easy reach of your bed. As soon as you wake up from a dream, jot down

---

[18] Ann Faraday, The Dream Game (New York: Harper & Row, 1974).

as many details as you can remember, including the setting, characters, emotions, and any specific events or symbols. Don't worry about analyzing the dream right away; the goal is to capture the raw content before it fades from memory.

Over time, you may notice patterns or recurring themes in your dreams that offer insights into your subconscious mind. You can use these insights to explore your inner thoughts and feelings, leading to greater self-awareness and personal growth.

Dream journaling can be a powerful tool for self-discovery and emotional healing. By regularly recording and reflecting on your dreams, you can unlock the mysteries of your subconscious mind and foster a deeper connection with your inner self.

Mood Tracking

The concept of mood and its impact on various aspects of life, including sleep, gained significant attention during the psychedelic era of the 1970s. This period was marked by a cultural shift towards self-exploration and a heightened interest in understanding human emotions and consciousness. While the era popularized the exploration of feelings, the scientific study of mood and its effects has a solid foundation in psychology.

Paul Ekman, a pioneering psychologist in the study of emotions, made significant contributions to our understanding of how emotions are expressed and perceived. His research on facial expressions and the universality of emotions has implications for understanding mood and its impact on behavior and well-being.[19]

---

[19] Paul Ekman, Emotions Revealed: Recognizing Faces and Feelings to Improve Communication and Emotional Life (New York: Times Books, 2003).

Martin Seligman, another influential psychologist, is known for his work on positive psychology and the concept of learned helplessness.[20] His research on optimism and well-being provides insights into how positive moods can enhance resilience and overall life satisfaction, which in turn can influence sleep quality.

The invention of mood rings in 1975 by Joshua Reynolds and Maris Ambats added a cultural artifact to the fascination with mood. These rings contained a heat-sensitive liquid crystal that changed color supposedly reflecting the wearer's mood. While the scientific accuracy of mood rings is debatable, they became a symbol of the era's interest in emotional awareness.

The relationship between mood and sleep has been explored in various studies. One such study examined the correlation between daily variability in sleep patterns and mood, highlighting the impact of mood on sleep quality and consistency.[21] Another relevant study evaluated the role of insomnia as a predictor of depression, further illustrating the bidirectional relationship between mood and sleep.[22] These studies, among others, provide evidence for the strong connection between mood and sleep, indicating that mood can

---

[20] Martin E.P. Seligman, Learned Optimism: How to Change Your Mind and Your Life (New York: Pocket Books, 1998).

[21] Bei, B., Wiley, J. F., Trinder, J., & Manber, R. (2016). Beyond the mean: A systematic review on the correlates of daily intraindividual variability in sleep/wake patterns. Sleep Medicine Reviews, 28, 108-124. https://doi.org/10.1016/j.smrv.2015.06.003

[22] Baglioni, C., Battagliese, G., Feige, B., Spiegelhalder, K., Nissen, C., Voderholzer, U., Lombardo, C., & Riemann, D. (2011). Insomnia as a predictor of depression: A meta-analytic evaluation of longitudinal epidemiological studies. Journal of Affective Disorders, 135(1-3), 10-19. https://doi.org/10.1016/j.jad.2011.01.011

significantly affect sleep quality and that sleep disturbances can impact mood.

A negative or bad mood, characterized by anxiety and stress, can activate the body's fight-or-flight response, making it difficult to relax and fall asleep. On the other hand, a positive or good mood can promote relaxation and increase the likelihood of restful sleep. Understanding and managing mood is crucial for maintaining healthy sleep patterns, and techniques like mood tracking as a relaxation exercise can be an effective tool for improving sleep quality.

Mood tracking may also be helpful for monitoring your emotional well-being and understanding how your mood and daily activities can impact your sleep quality. By keeping a record of your emotions and the events of your day, you can identify patterns and triggers that may be affecting your ability to fall asleep or stay asleep.

To start mood tracking, you can use a journal, a mobile app, or a simple chart to record your mood at different times throughout the day. Alongside your mood, note any significant activities, events, or interactions that may have influenced how you felt. This can include work-related tasks, social engagements, exercise, meals, and any other experiences that stand out.

Over time, you may begin to notice correlations between your mood and certain activities or events. For example, you might find that on days when you exercise, your mood improves and you sleep better at night. Alternatively, you may notice that stressful work meetings lead to a decrease in mood and difficulty sleeping.

By identifying these patterns, you can make informed lifestyle changes to enhance your sleep quality. For instance, if you discover that caffeine consumption in the afternoon negatively impacts your sleep, you can adjust your habits to avoid caffeine later in the day. Similarly, if you find that engaging in relaxing activities before bed, such as reading or taking a warm bath, improves your mood and sleep, you can incorporate these practices into your nightly routine.

Mood tracking can also help you recognize when you may need to seek professional support for mental health issues that could be affecting your sleep, such as anxiety or depression. By monitoring your mood and its impact on your sleep, you can take proactive steps to address any underlying issues and improve your overall well-being.

Setting Intentions

The practice of setting intentions has its roots in various spiritual and philosophical traditions, including yoga. In yoga philosophy, the concept of intention is closely associated with the Sanskrit term "sankalpa." Sankalpa can be translated as a vow or a resolve, and it represents a commitment to align one's actions with one's deepest values and desires.

Setting intentions or sankalpas is a way to bring focus and clarity to one's aspirations, helping to direct energy and attention toward desired outcomes. By consciously choosing and affirming one's intentions, individuals can create a sense of purpose and direction, both on and off the yoga mat.

The practice of setting intentions has been embraced in various modern self-help and personal development contexts, extending beyond the realm of yoga. It is seen as a powerful tool for manifesting goals, fostering personal growth, and cultivating a mindful approach to life. Setting intentions can be a transformative practice that helps individuals align their actions with their values and aspirations.

In the realm of personal development and manifestation, gurus like Bob Proctor have championed the practice of setting intentions as a fundamental principle for achieving success and fulfillment.[23] These experts argue that by clearly defining and focusing on our intentions, we harness the power of our subconscious mind to attract the experiences and outcomes we desire. They emphasize the importance of not only setting intentions, but also maintaining a positive mindset and a strong belief in the possibility of achieving these goals.

This approach is often linked to the Law of Attraction, which suggests that like attracts like, and by emitting positive energy through our intentions, we can attract positive results. In a sense combining the practice of setting intentions with visualization techniques, affirmations, and consistent action, in some instances may lead effectively to manifesting goals to create a life that aligns more closely with our deepest aspirations. This principle of intentional living and manifestation has become a cornerstone in the teachings of many modern self-help and personal development experts, offering a powerful tool for personal transformation and growth.

As such setting intentions before going to bed can be a powerful practice that can help you end your day with a sense of purpose and clarity. By taking a few moments to write down your intentions or goals for the next day, you create a roadmap for what you wish to achieve, which can provide a sense of direction and focus.

This practice can be particularly beneficial for sleep because it helps to quiet the mind. When you have a clear plan for the next

---

[23] Bob Proctor, You Were Born Rich (Scottsdale, AZ: LifeSuccess Productions, 1984).

day, you're less likely to lie in bed worrying about what needs to be done or feeling overwhelmed by tasks. Instead, you can go to bed feeling prepared and organized, which can foster a more peaceful state of mind and make it easier to fall asleep.

Setting intentions also allows you to prioritize your activities and ensure that your actions align with your values and long-term goals. This can increase your sense of control and satisfaction, reducing stress and anxiety, which are common barriers to restful sleep.

To incorporate this practice into your bedtime routine, keep a notebook or journal by your bed. Before turning off the lights, take a few minutes to reflect on what you want to accomplish the next day. Write down a few specific, achievable goals or intentions. These could range from completing a work project to practicing self-care or spending quality time with family.

By setting intentions before sleep, you not only enhance your sleep quality but also set the stage for a productive and fulfilling day ahead. This practice can be a simple yet effective way to improve your overall well-being and ensure that you wake up feeling focused and ready to tackle the day.

Positive Affirmations

The concept of affirmations has gained significant popularity over the years, becoming a widely recognized tool for personal development and success. At the forefront of this movement is Napoleon Hill, whose work has had a profound impact on the popularization of affirmations. In 1937, Hill published his seminal book, "Think and Grow Rich," which has since become a classic in the self-help genre.[24] In this book, Hill outlines the principles of success he uncovered through interviewing over 500 successful men. One of the key concepts he introduced was the power of affirmations—positive statements that, when repeated regularly, can influence the subconscious mind and propel individuals toward their goals.

The use of affirmations has not been limited to business moguls and entrepreneurs; it has also found its way into the routines of many celebrities. Jennifer Lawrence, for example, has spoken about using affirmations to boost her confidence and self-esteem, particularly in the face of the pressures of Hollywood. Oprah Winfrey, a well-known proponent of personal growth and self-improvement, has also shared how affirmations have played a role in her success. Similarly, the singer Rihanna has credited affirmations with helping her maintain a positive mindset and overcome challenges.

The appeal of affirmations lies in their simplicity and accessibility. By focusing on positive, empowering statements, individuals can shift their mindset, overcome self-doubt, and create a more positive outlook on life. As more people, including celebrities, share their experiences with affirmations, their popularity continues to grow, making them a staple in the toolkit of personal development.

Positive affirmations are powerful statements that can help shift your mindset and promote a sense of peace and well-being, especially before sleep. By focusing on positive affirmations, you can reprogram your subconscious mind to let go of negative thoughts and embrace a more optimistic outlook, which can be particularly beneficial for improving sleep quality.

---

[24] Hill, Napoleon. Think and Grow Rich. The Ralston Society, 1937.

Writing down positive affirmations before bed allows you to end your day on a positive note. You can create affirmations that specifically address any anxieties or worries that might interfere with your sleep. For example, if you often find yourself stressed about the next day's tasks, you might write an affirmation like, "I am prepared for tomorrow and trust that everything will unfold perfectly."

Reading these affirmations before turning off the lights can help calm your mind and set the tone for a restful night. You can keep a list of affirmations by your bedside and read them aloud or silently to yourself. This practice helps reinforce the positive messages, making it easier for your mind to relax and let go of any lingering stress.

Positive affirmations for sleep might include statements like the following.

"I release all worries and embrace a peaceful sleep."

"My body and mind are relaxed and ready for rest."

"I am grateful for this day and look forward to a rejuvenating night's sleep."

"Each breath I take fills me with calm and serenity."

"I am surrounded by love and positivity, ensuring a restful sleep."

“I am grateful for this day and ready to embrace a restful sleep.”

“My mind is calm, and my body is relaxed, preparing for a deep sleep.”

“I release all tension and stress from the day, allowing myself to drift into peaceful slumber.”

“Each breath I take fills me with relaxation and tranquility.”

"I am safe and secure, allowing myself to let go and fall asleep peacefully."

"My bedroom is a sanctuary for rest, and I am surrounded by comfort and peace."

"I trust in my body's ability to restore itself during sleep, waking up refreshed and energized."

"I let go of all worries and concerns, knowing that tomorrow is a new day."

"I welcome sleep with open arms, grateful for the restorative power it brings."

"As I close my eyes, I invite peace and calmness to envelop me, guiding me into a night of deep, rejuvenating sleep."

By incorporating positive affirmations into your bedtime routine, you can create a nurturing environment for your mind and body. This practice can help you shift away from negative thought patterns and embrace a more positive state, making it easier to fall asleep and enjoy a deeper, more restorative sleep.

Sleep Analysis

Sleep analysis involves keeping a detailed record of your sleep patterns to gain insights into your sleep habits and identify areas for improvement. By tracking when you go to bed, how long it takes you to fall asleep, the number of times you wake up during the night, and the time you wake up in the morning, you can begin to understand the quality and quantity of your sleep. This information can be invaluable in identifying trends or habits that may be impacting your sleep, such as the effects of caffeine or screen time before bed, or the influence of stress and anxiety on your ability to sleep through the night.

The history and origin of sleep analysis can be traced back to the pioneering work of Nathaniel Kleitman, often referred to as the "father of modern sleep research." Kleitman's groundbreaking contributions laid the foundation for our understanding of sleep and its various stages.

In 1925, Kleitman published his first major work, "Sleep and Wakefulness," which was one of the earliest systematic studies of sleep.[25] His research was instrumental in establishing sleep as a distinct and important area of scientific investigation. Kleitman's work was characterized by his meticulous approach to studying sleep patterns and his innovative use of technology to monitor physiological changes during sleep.

One of Kleitman's most significant contributions to the field was the establishment of the world's first sleep laboratory at the University of Chicago in 1957. This laboratory became a hub for sleep research, attracting scientists from around the world and facilitating numerous groundbreaking studies. In collaboration with Allan Rechtschaffen, Professor Emeritus of Psychology, Psychiatry, and the College at the University of Chicago, Kleitman conducted extensive research on sleep disorders, sleep deprivation, and the structure of sleep.

Their collaboration led to the discovery of rapid eye movement (REM) sleep, a finding that revolutionized the field of sleep research. REM sleep, characterized by rapid eye movements, increased brain activity, and vivid dreaming, is now recognized as a

---

[25] Kleitman, Nathaniel. Sleep and Wakefulness. University of Chicago Press, 1963.

critical component of the sleep cycle. The formal classification of these stages by Allan Rechtschaffen and Anthony Kales in the 1960s further advanced the field, providing a framework for studying sleep patterns and disorders.[26]

The legacy of Nathaniel Kleitman and his work at the University of Chicago continues to influence the field of sleep research. His pioneering efforts have paved the way for a deeper understanding of the complexities of sleep and its impact on human health and well-being.

The field of sleep analysis has experienced significant breakthroughs that have deepened our understanding of sleep and its impact on human health. Research into circadian rhythms, the internal biological clocks regulating sleep-wake cycles, has also been instrumental in understanding sleep. Franz Halberg's work in the 20th century on circadian rhythms shed light on how these natural cycles influence sleep and overall health.[27] This research has implications for managing sleep disorders and optimizing sleep schedules to align with our biological clocks.

Advancements in technology, such as polysomnography and neuroimaging tools like EEG and fMRI, have enabled scientists to explore the brain's activity during sleep with greater precision. These tools have unveiled the complex neural mechanisms underlying sleep and its various stages, leading to a more comprehensive understanding of sleep's role in cognitive and emotional regulation.

---

[26] Rechtschaffen, Allan, and Anthony Kales, eds. A Manual of Standardized Terminology, Techniques and Scoring System for Sleep Stages of Human Subjects. UCLA Brain Information Service/Brain Research Institute, 1968.

[27] Halberg, Franz. "Chronobiology: Methodological Problems." Acta Medica Scandinavica, vol. 180, no. S678, 1966, pp. 1-10.

Additionally, the establishment of the International Classification of Sleep Disorders by the American Academy of Sleep Medicine has improved the diagnosis and treatment of conditions such as insomnia, sleep apnea, and narcolepsy, enhancing the quality of life for those affected by sleep-related issues.

Overall, the breakthroughs in sleep analysis have not only expanded our knowledge of the fundamental nature of sleep but also paved the way for more effective interventions and treatments for sleep-related disorders, highlighting the importance of sleep in maintaining physical and mental well-being.

While professional sleep studies in a lab with sensors, wires, and EEG caps provide comprehensive insights, you don't necessarily need such extensive setups for basic sleep analysis. You can conduct a simple DIY sleep analysis with just a pen, paper, and some self-reflection. By keeping a sleep diary, you can track your bedtime, wake-up time, sleep duration, and any disturbances during the night. This self-monitoring can help you identify patterns and habits affecting your sleep quality. Reflecting on your daily activities, caffeine intake, and stress levels can also provide valuable insights into how your lifestyle influences your sleep. This DIY approach is a practical and accessible way to start understanding your sleep patterns and making informed changes for better rest.

Here's an example of a sleep analysis journal entry to show how you can write a quick overview of the night's sleep to help track details about bedtime routines, sleep disturbances, and factors that might have influenced sleep quality. Regular entries like this can help identify patterns and areas for improvement in sleep habits.

***

Date: January 18, 2024

Bedtime: 11:00 PM

Time to Fall Asleep: Approximately 20 minutes

Night Awakenings:

- 2:30 AM (Awake for 10 minutes, bathroom break)
- 4:45 AM (Awake for 5 minutes, unknown reason)

Wake-up Time: 7:00 AM

Total Sleep Time: 7 hours 25 minutes

Sleep Quality (1-10): 7

Dream Recall: Had a vivid dream about being on a beach vacation.

Evening Activities Before Bed:

- 9:00 PM: Light exercise (yoga)
- 10:00 PM: Read a book for 30 minutes
- 10:45 PM: Turned off all screens, dimmed the lights

Daytime Factors:

- Moderate stress level at work
- Consumed 2 cups of coffee in the morning, none after 2 PM
- Felt moderately tired throughout the day

Notes:

- Felt relatively relaxed before bed due to yoga session.
- Waking up at 4:45 AM was unusual; no apparent reason. Might need to monitor if this continues.

***

Over time, sleep analysis can help you make informed decisions about changes you may need to make to your sleep routine or environment. For example, you might discover that you sleep better on nights when you engage in a relaxing bedtime routine or that you struggle to fall asleep when you eat a heavy meal too close to bedtime. By making adjustments based on your sleep analysis, you can work towards achieving more restful and restorative sleep, which is crucial for your overall health and well-being.

Additionally, sleep analysis can also be useful in identifying potential sleep disorders, such as insomnia or sleep apnea. If you notice persistent patterns of disrupted sleep or difficulty falling or staying asleep, it may be a sign to consult a healthcare professional for further evaluation and treatment.

Letter Writing

The practice of writing letters to express and process emotions has a long history, with roots that can be traced back to various cultures and periods. One notable historical figure who utilized this method was Abraham Lincoln, the 16th President of the United States. Lincoln was known for writing "hot letters" when he was angry or upset. These letters were a way for him to vent his frustrations and articulate his feelings without causing immediate conflict. Instead of sending these letters, Lincoln would set them aside until his emotions had cooled down, often marking them with "Never sent. Never signed." This practice allowed him to revisit his thoughts with a clearer mind the next day, providing perspective and preventing rash decisions.[28]

[28] "The Value Of The Unsent Angry Letter." NPR, 6 June 2014, www.npr.org/2014/06/06/319420036/the-value-of-the-unsent-angry-letter.

The concept of writing letters to manage emotions, sometimes referred to as "the lost art of the unsent angry letter" or a "Lincoln letter," highlights the therapeutic power of writing. By putting thoughts and feelings into words, sometimes we can gain clarity, release pent-up emotions, and reflect on our experiences. This practice can be particularly useful in situations where direct communication is not possible or advisable, allowing for a private space to process emotions.

In modern times, the idea of writing letters for emotional release has evolved into various forms, including journaling and expressive writing. These practices are often recommended by mental health professionals as a way to cope with stress, anxiety, and other emotional challenges. Writing letters, whether they are intended to be sent or not, provides a structured way to explore and express feelings, leading to emotional catharsis and a deeper understanding of oneself.

Letter writing can be a powerful tool for emotional release, especially when dealing with feelings of frustration, anger, or hurt caused by a situation or person. The act of writing a letter allows you to express your emotions in a safe and controlled environment, without the immediate consequences of direct confrontation. This exercise can be particularly therapeutic when it involves the concept of forgiveness.

Forgiveness is a crucial aspect of emotional healing and personal growth. Holding onto resentment and anger can be emotionally draining and can even have negative impacts on physical health. Writing a letter is a way to practice forgiveness, even if you're not ready to express it directly to the person involved. In the letter, you can articulate your feelings, acknowledge the pain caused, and express a willingness to move past the hurt. This doesn't mean you're condoning the behavior or forgetting what happened, but rather you're choosing to let go of the bitterness for your own well-being.

The beauty of this exercise is that you don't have to send the letter. The purpose is not to elicit a response or to provoke the other person but to provide yourself with a sense of closure and emotional release. It's a private, personal way to work through your feelings and to come to terms with them. If you do choose to send the letter, it can be a step towards reconciliation, but that's not a necessary outcome.

Here's an example of a "hot letter."

***

Dear Jack,

I'm writing this letter to express my feelings about some of the interactions we've had recently. I've noticed several instances where your comments and behavior felt condescending and dismissive. For example, when you said, "You're not as slow as you look," it came across as quite patronizing. In the moment, I was taken aback and didn't respond, but I wish I had said, "Gee, was that a hint of condescension I detected? How about we dial down the sass a notch?"

These microaggressions are not only uncomfortable, but they also have a significant impact on my self-esteem and performance. I find myself second-guessing my abilities and contributions, which I know is not conducive to a productive work environment. Moreover, such behavior doesn't just affect me; it creates an unwelcoming atmosphere for everyone involved. It's disheartening to see how these subtle forms of discrimination can perpetuate a cycle of inequality and hinder progress.

I've also noticed that these incidents have been affecting me outside of work. I find myself replaying these interactions in my head, losing sleep over what I could have said or done differently. It's frustrating to feel like I'm being held back not by my capabilities, but by an environment that allows these microaggressions to go unchecked.

I'm writing this letter not to point fingers or create conflict, but to bring awareness to how these seemingly small actions can have a profound impact on individuals and the workplace as a whole. I hope that we can work towards a more respectful and inclusive environment where everyone feels valued and supported.

Right now, I'm taking a deep breath and forgiving you for your words, and forgiving myself for letting them hurt. I am releasing and letting go, knowing in my heart that with this small act we'll both do better, and allowing myself to release these thoughts and fall asleep.

Sincerely,

Your Co-Worker and Friend

***

In summary, writing a letter to express your feelings, especially when incorporating the concept of forgiveness, can be a cathartic experience. It allows you to confront your emotions, articulate them clearly, and work towards letting go of negative feelings. This exercise can be a valuable step in the journey towards emotional healing and personal growth.

In conclusion, relaxation exercises play a crucial role in promoting better sleep and overall well-being. Techniques such as deep breathing, progressive muscle relaxation, visualization, and writing "hot letters" offer effective ways to unwind, release tension, and quiet the mind before bedtime. By incorporating these exercises into your nightly routine, you can create a conducive environment for restful sleep, improve sleep quality, and enhance your ability to cope with stress and emotions. Remember, the key to success with these exercises is consistency and personalization. Find what works best for you, and make it a regular part of your sleep hygiene to enjoy the benefits of a more relaxed mind and body, leading to a more restorative and rejuvenating night's sleep.

16

Natural Remedies For Better Sleep

For many, the sweet surrender to slumber remains elusive, a treasure just beyond reach. This chapter looks at natural remedies for those seeking better sleep. We explore the soothing symphony of foods that whisper lullabies to our nervous system, from magnesium-rich foods like leafy greens to the gentle tryptophan effects of turkey. Sips of serenity await in night-time teas, with chamomile's calming caress and valerian's sedative melody. Movement, too, plays its part—through the graceful dance of yoga or the rhythmic lull of an evening stroll, our bodies are coaxed toward a state of restful readiness. A harmony of lifestyle choices can guide restless sleepers towards the restorative sanctuary of better sleep—naturally.

Food and Drink

Certain foods and drinks are believed to have properties that may help improve sleep quality. Here are some natural substances and their potential sleep-promoting effects:

Chamomile Tea:

Why it might help: Chamomile contains apigenin, an antioxidant that binds to certain receptors in the brain that may promote sleepiness and reduce insomnia.

Tart Cherry Juice:

Why it might help: Tart cherries are a natural source of melatonin, a hormone that regulates sleep. Some studies suggest that consuming tart cherry juice may improve sleep quality and duration.

Valerian Root:

Examples: Valerian root tea, valerian root capsules, valerian root tinctures, and valerian root extracts.

Why it might help: Valerian root has been used for centuries as a remedy for various ailments, including sleep disorders. Some studies suggest it may help improve sleep quality and reduce the time it takes to fall asleep.

Lavender:

Examples: Lavender essential oil (for aromatherapy), lavender-infused pillows or sachets, lavender tea.

Why it might help: While typically inhaled or used topically, lavender's calming properties are well-known. Consuming lavender as a tea or in other edible forms might have similar relaxing effects, though more research is needed.

Warm Milk:

Why it might help: It's believed that warm milk may increase levels of tryptophan in the blood, which the body can convert to melatonin. The psychological comfort of drinking warm milk might also promote relaxation.

Bananas:

Why it might help: Bananas are a good source of magnesium and potassium. Both minerals act as muscle relaxants, potentially promoting sleep.

Magnesium-rich Foods:

Examples: Almonds, spinach, and cashews.

Why they might help: Magnesium may improve sleep quality, especially for those with insomnia, by helping to relax the muscles and calm the nervous system.

Omega-3 Fatty Acids:

Examples: Fatty fish like salmon, mackerel, and sardines.

Why they might help: Omega-3 fatty acids, particularly DHA, may boost the production of serotonin, a sleep-enhancing brain chemical.

Kiwi:

Why it might help: Some studies suggest that kiwi's antioxidant properties and its serotonin content can improve sleep onset, duration, and efficiency.

Vitamin B:

Examples: For Vitamin B6 - bananas, chickpeas, and tuna; for Vitamin B12 - beef, eggs, and fortified cereals; for Folate (B9) - spinach, asparagus, and brussels sprouts. Vitamin B is also commonly found in multivitamins and B-complex supplements.

Why it might help: Vitamin B plays a significant role in promoting better sleep, primarily through its influence on the nervous system and the regulation of certain hormones and neurotransmitters that are crucial for sleep.

Passionflower:

Examples: Passionflower tea, passionflower extract supplements.

Why it might help: Passionflower is believed to have calming effects, which can help reduce anxiety and improve sleep quality. It is thought to increase levels of gamma-aminobutyric acid (GABA) in the brain, a chemical that reduces brain activity and promotes relaxation.

Melatonin-Inducing Foods:

Examples: Cherries, walnuts, and bananas.

Why they might help: Melatonin is a hormone that regulates the sleep-wake cycle. Foods that are rich in melatonin or that promote its production can help to improve sleep onset and quality. For instance, cherries are one of the few natural food sources of melatonin, while bananas contain tryptophan, an amino acid that the body uses to produce melatonin.

Glycine:

Examples: Bone broth, meat, fish, and soy products.

Why it might help: Glycine is an amino acid that may improve sleep quality by lowering body temperature and promoting relaxation. Taking glycine before bed has been shown to help people fall asleep faster and achieve deeper, more restful sleep.

Cannabidiol (CBD):

Examples: CBD oil, CBD capsules, and CBD-infused edibles.

Why it might help: CBD is a compound found in cannabis that has been shown to have calming and anxiety-reducing effects. Unlike its counterpart THC, CBD does not produce psychoactive effects. It may help improve sleep by reducing anxiety and promoting relaxation, though more research is needed to fully understand its effects on sleep.

5-HTP (5-Hydroxytryptophan):

Examples: Supplements derived from the seeds of the African plant Griffonia simplicifolia.

Why it might help: 5-HTP is a precursor to serotonin, a neurotransmitter that plays a key role in mood and sleep regulation. By increasing serotonin levels, 5-HTP may help improve sleep quality, especially in individuals with sleep disorders or depression.

Kava:

Examples: Kava tea, kava supplements, and kava extract.

Why it might help: Kava is a plant native to the South Pacific islands known for its calming and sedative effects. It is believed to work by affecting neurotransmitter levels in the brain, including GABA, which promotes relaxation and can aid in sleep.

Hops:

Examples: Hops supplements, hops tea, and as an ingredient in some sleep-promoting herbal blends.

Why it might help: Hops, a key ingredient in beer, have natural sedative properties and have been used traditionally to promote relaxation and sleep. They are believed to work by increasing GABA activity in the brain, which helps induce sleep.

Ashwagandha:

Examples: Ashwagandha supplements, ashwagandha powder, and ashwagandha tea.

Why it might help: Ashwagandha is an adaptogenic herb used in Ayurvedic medicine to help reduce stress and anxiety, which can in turn improve sleep quality. It is believed to work by regulating the body's stress response and promoting relaxation.

GABA (Gamma-Aminobutyric Acid):

Examples: GABA supplements and GABA-enriched foods such as fermented products like kimchi, miso, and tempeh.

Why it might help: GABA is a neurotransmitter that inhibits neural activity, promoting relaxation and reducing anxiety. Supplementing with GABA may help improve sleep by calming the nervous system and making it easier to fall asleep.

Ginkgo Biloba:

Examples: Ginkgo biloba supplements, ginkgo biloba tea, and ginkgo biloba extract.

Why it might help: Ginkgo biloba is believed to have a positive effect on sleep by reducing stress and improving relaxation. It may also help regulate sleep patterns by improving blood circulation and oxygen flow to the brain. However, more research is needed to fully understand its impact on sleep.

Turkey Dinner:

Examples: A traditional Thanksgiving meal with roasted turkey, stuffing, mashed potatoes, and gravy.

Why it might help: Turkey is known for its high content of tryptophan, an amino acid that is a precursor to serotonin, a neurotransmitter that can be converted into the hormone melatonin. Melatonin is involved in regulating the sleep-wake cycle. Additionally, the consumption of a large meal, such as a turkey dinner, can lead to a feeling of fullness and drowsiness, which may also contribute to sleepiness.

Turkey Tail:

Examples: Turkey tail mushroom tea, turkey tail mushroom supplements, and turkey tail mushroom extracts.

Why it might help: While it's not like eating a Turkey dinner, Turkey tail mushrooms contain polysaccharides, which can have a sedative effect, potentially promoting relaxation and improving sleep quality. They are also rich in beta-glucans, which are known for their immune-boosting properties which may support overall health, contributing to a more restful sleep.

Reishi:

Examples: Reishi mushroom tea, reishi mushroom supplements, and reishi mushroom extracts.

Why it might help: Reishi mushrooms, also known as Ganoderma lucidum, are believed to have adaptogenic properties that can help reduce stress and promote relaxation, which may improve sleep quality. They are thought to work by modulating the immune system and affecting the levels of certain neurotransmitters in the brain.

Chaga:

Examples: Chaga mushroom tea, chaga mushroom supplements, and chaga mushroom extracts.

Why it might help: Chaga mushrooms are known for their high antioxidant content and potential immune-boosting properties. While there is limited research on chaga's direct effects on sleep, its potential to reduce inflammation and support overall health may indirectly contribute to better sleep quality by promoting a more relaxed and balanced state in the body.

It's essential to consider the timing of consumption. Eating or drinking large amounts right before bed can cause discomfort or indigestion, which can hinder sleep. Small portions or a cup of a calming beverage is usually more appropriate. It's important to remember that everyone's body is different. What works for one person might not work for another.

While these foods and drinks may aid sleep, they're just one piece of the puzzle. Good sleep hygiene, including a consistent sleep schedule, a comfortable sleep environment, and relaxation techniques, also play significant roles in achieving deep, restorative sleep.

Temperature

Maintaining a cool temperature during sleep is increasingly recognized as a key factor in improving sleep quality. The concept is based on the body's natural circadian rhythm, which favors a cooler environment for deep, restorative sleep. By using products that regulate bed temperature, individuals can mitigate the heat buildup that occurs under covers and in modern beds with foam materials.

The science behind this approach is rooted in the understanding that our bodies are designed to cool down during sleep. A drop in core body temperature by about two degrees is optimal for entering deep sleep, a phase crucial for physical and mental recovery. Adjustable temperature settings allow users to find their ideal sleeping environment, ranging from 55 to 78 degrees Fahrenheit, depending on personal preference. According to Tara Young, the ideal sleep temperature most restful for older adults is between 68° and 77° Fahrenheit.[29]

The benefits of maintaining a cool sleeping environment extend beyond just the individual sleeper. Couples with different temperature preferences can each find comfort with adjustable settings, promoting better sleep for both partners. This can lead to improved mood, cognitive function, and overall well-being.

Interestingly, the preference for a cooler sleeping environment may have evolutionary roots. Early humans, or cave people, likely evolved to sleep better on the cold ground, as cooler temperatures would have been a natural part of their sleeping environment. This adaptation may have carried over into modern humans, underscoring the importance of cool temperatures for optimal sleep.

In summary, harnessing the power of cool temperatures during sleep is a simple yet effective solution for enhancing sleep quality, making it a valuable addition to anyone's sleep routine.

Activities

Activities before bedtime can significantly influence the quality of sleep. Here's a breakdown of some common pre-bedtime activities and their potential effects on sleep:

---

[29] Young, Tara. "Finding Your Ideal Sleep Temperature." ChiliSleep Blog, 23 July 2021, www.chilisleep.com/blogs/news/ideal-sleep-temperature.

Exercise:

Effect: Moderate exercise earlier in the day can promote deeper sleep and reduce the time it takes to fall asleep. However, vigorous exercise too close to bedtime can be stimulating and potentially disrupt sleep.

Recommendation: Aim for regular exercise but try to finish any vigorous workouts at least 2-3 hours before bedtime.

Going to the Bathroom:

Effect: Emptying your bladder before bed can prevent disruptions during the night, leading to more uninterrupted and deeper sleep.

Recommendation: Make it a habit to visit the bathroom right before going to bed.

Sex:

Effect: Sex releases oxytocin (the "love hormone") and reduces cortisol (a stress-related hormone), which can promote relaxation and better sleep.

Recommendation: If conducive to relaxation and sleep, incorporating intimacy as a regular part of one's bedtime routine can be beneficial.

Reduced Screen Time (Phones, Tablets, Computers):

Effect: The blue light emitted by screens can interfere with the production of melatonin, a hormone that regulates sleep.

Recommendation: Reduce screen time at least an hour before bed or use "night mode" settings that decrease blue light exposure.

Reduced TV Watching:

Effect: Similar to other screens, the blue light from TVs can disrupt melatonin production. The content of what's being watched can also be stimulating or anxiety-provoking.

Recommendation: Choose calming programs and reduce brightness or use a blue light filter if possible. Limit TV watching in the hour leading up to bedtime.

Reading:

Effect: Reading can be a calming activity for many, especially when using traditional books. However, reading suspenseful or anxiety-inducing material can have the opposite effect.

Recommendation: Opt for calming or neutral reading material before bed. If using an e-reader, ensure it's not emitting disruptive blue light.

Taking a Bath:

Effect: A warm bath or shower can help relax the muscles and lower cortisol levels. The drop in body temperature after getting out of the bath can also signal to the body that it's time to sleep.

Recommendation: Taking a warm bath 1-2 hours before bedtime can be beneficial for sleep.

Meditation or Deep Breathing:

Effect: These relaxation techniques can reduce anxiety, calm the mind, and prepare the body for rest.

Recommendation: Incorporating a short meditation or deep breathing routine before bed can enhance sleep quality.

Reduced Alcohol Consumption:

Effect: While alcohol might make individuals feel sleepy initially, it can interrupt the sleep cycle, reducing the quality of sleep.

Recommendation: Limit alcohol consumption, especially close to bedtime.

Avoid Eating Heavy Meals:

Effect: Eating a large or heavy meal before bed can lead to discomfort and indigestion, disrupting sleep.

Recommendation: Finish eating at least 2-3 hours before bedtime and avoid heavy, rich foods.

It's essential to recognize that individual reactions to these activities can vary. What works well for one person might not work for another, so observing one's patterns and adjusting bedtime routines accordingly is crucial.

Interventions

Sleep is influenced by a myriad of factors, ranging from our environment to our daily habits. While many activities and interventions can enhance sleep quality, some tend to have a more significant impact across a broader spectrum of individuals. Here are some key interventions that generally make the most difference:

Consistent Sleep Schedule:

Impact: Going to bed and waking up at the same time every day, even on weekends, helps regulate the body's internal clock and improves the consistency of sleep.

Sleep Environment:

Impact: A dark, quiet, and cool room generally promotes better sleep. Factors like comfortable mattresses and pillows, as well as eliminating light and noise pollution, can make a substantial difference in sleep quality.

Limiting Blue Light Exposure:

Impact: Exposure to blue light from screens (phones, tablets, computers, TVs) before bedtime can significantly reduce melatonin production, thus hindering sleep.

Mindfulness and Relaxation Techniques:

Impact: Practices like deep breathing, meditation, and progressive muscle relaxation can reduce anxiety and induce a state of calm, making it easier to fall and stay asleep.

Limiting Caffeine and Alcohol:

Impact: Both substances can interfere with the sleep cycle. While caffeine can keep you awake, alcohol can reduce the quality of sleep.

Regular Physical Activity:

Impact: Regular exercise can help regulate sleep patterns and increase the duration of deep sleep. However, timing matters, as exercising too close to bedtime can be stimulating.

Diet:

Impact: Consuming large or spicy meals can cause discomfort and indigestion. On the other hand, certain foods and drinks, like chamomile tea or magnesium-rich foods, can potentially promote sleep.

Managing Stress and Anxiety:

Impact: Chronic stress or unresolved anxiety can significantly disrupt sleep. Adopting coping strategies, such as journaling, therapy, or other stress-reducing techniques, can lead to better sleep over time.

Limiting Naps:

Impact: While naps can be beneficial, especially if they're short and not too late in the day, long or irregular napping can negatively affect sleep.

Establishing a Bedtime Routine:

Impact: Engaging in relaxing activities before bed, such as reading, taking a warm bath, or listening to soothing music, can signal to your body that it's time to wind down.

Out of these, the importance can vary for different individuals based on personal habits, health conditions, and lifestyle. But often, maintaining a consistent sleep schedule, optimizing the sleep environment, managing blue light exposure, and managing stress are among the top influencers for most people.

Regardless of the interventions you choose, consistency is vital. Establishing and maintaining good sleep habits over the long term often yields the most substantial benefits.

Newborn Sleep Tips for New Parents

Sleep strategies for newborns are notably different from those for adults. The sleep patterns and needs of infants are unique to their developmental stage. Here are some recommended techniques and practices to promote better sleep for newborns:

Swaddling:

Why: Swaddling can mimic the snugness of the womb, providing a familiar and comforting environment for newborns. It can also prevent involuntary reflexes that might startle the baby awake.

Note: Ensure you know how to swaddle safely. The baby's face should be clear of any fabric, and the swaddle shouldn't be too tight, especially around the hips.

White Noise:

Why: White noise machines or apps can replicate the constant sounds the baby heard in the womb, providing a calming and familiar auditory environment.

Pacifiers:

Why: Sucking can be soothing for babies. For some infants, a pacifier can be calming and help them fall asleep.

Note: Introduce a pacifier after breastfeeding has been well-established if you're nursing.

Room-Sharing:

Why: The American Academy of Pediatrics (AAP) recommends room-sharing (baby sleeps in the same room but on a separate sleep surface) for at least the first six months. This can make nighttime feedings easier and has been shown to reduce the risk of SIDS (Sudden Infant Death Syndrome).

Dark and Quiet Environment:

Why: While newborns can sleep through a fair amount of noise and light, a dim, quiet room can help establish a night-day rhythm and improve sleep as they age.

Consistent Bedtime Routine:

Why: Even in the early weeks, establishing a simple, consistent bedtime routine can signal to your baby that it's time to sleep. This might include activities like a warm bath, a lullaby, or reading a short story.

Feeding Before Sleep:

Why: A full belly can help a newborn sleep longer stretches at a time. This is often why many parents opt for a "dream feed" right before they go to bed themselves.

Avoiding Overstimulation:

Why: Too much activity or stimulation right before bed can make it harder for a baby to settle down.

Recognizing Sleep Cues:

Why: Newborns often show signs when they're tired, such as fussing, yawning, or rubbing their eyes. Recognizing and acting on these cues promptly can make it easier to put the baby down.

Safe Sleep Environment:

Why: Always place your baby on their back to sleep, on a firm sleep surface without pillows, blankets, or soft toys. This reduces the risk of SIDS.

Baby Massage:

Why: Gentle massage can relax your baby and can be a soothing part of the bedtime routine.

It's important to remember that every baby is unique, and what works for one may not work for another.

It can take time and experimentation to figure out the best routines and techniques. Lastly, while these strategies can promote longer sleep stretches, it's natural for newborns to wake frequently in the night, especially in the early weeks and months.

17

Conclusion

In the quiet hours of the night when the world is still, the quest for a peaceful slumber seems paramount. In this practice of Mindful Slumber we journey through the gentle cadences of guided meditation, introducing the transformative power of mindfulness as a gateway to deeper, more restful sleep. As with any symphony, each component - from the serene guidance of meditation to the harmonious lullaby of the acoustic guitar, enriched by the healing resonance of 528 Hz binaural beats - plays its part in crafting an experience of holistic rest.

While this guide presents a singular meditation technique, its impact can be profound. It's a testament to the idea that sometimes, simplicity holds the key to unlocking our deepest desires—in this case, a night of undisturbed rest. The inclusion of the tranquil lullaby serves as a gentle reminder of the age-old connection between music and the mind, a connection enhanced further by the subtle, yet influential, binaural beats.

As you continue on your journey beyond these pages, may the insights and practices you've embraced serve as a comforting companion during restless nights. Remember that in the vast expanse of the universe, there lies a special frequency, a particular rhythm, attuned to your unique being. And every time you embark on this meditative voyage complemented by the strains of the guitar, you align closer to this personal symphony of serenity. Sleep, after all, is not just a nightly ritual, but a dance of the soul—a dance that "Mindful Slumber" hopes you'll cherish and master, night after tranquil night.

Good night and pleasant dreams.

www.ingramcontent.com/pod-product-compliance
Lightning Source LLC
Chambersburg PA
CBHW051302250726
48656CB00004B/1440

* 9 7 9 8 3 2 8 2 1 9 1 4 3 *